Breaking the
Cancer Code

Dearest Angel
~ Central ~
Thanks for growing
this project with
your love, support and
story. (page 121)
Yours in Health
Carolyn
8/22/13

Breaking the Cancer Code

A Revolutionary Approach to
Reversing Cancer

Geronimo Rubio MD and
Carolyn Gross

Library of Congress Control Number:		2013911553
ISBN:	Hardcover	978-1-4836-6048-6
	Softcover	978-1-4836-6047-9
	Ebook	978-1-4836-6049-3

Rev. date: 07/26/2013

To order additional copies of this book, contact:
Xlibris LLC
1-888-795-4274
www.Xlibris.com
Orders@Xlibris.com
131702

Contents

Preface

People respond deeply . . . to those who know what they stand for.

Dr. Geronimo Rubio's Story

I always felt like my life was destined for something good; it just started out that way. My father was a CPA and a very educated man. He would constantly reinforce that I was different, and he told my family, "My son was born with a guiding star!" I will always remember my father's words because he was telling me that I must look for the path less traveled to find my answers.

Significant moments and family stories define us. When I was eight years old, I was playing in my backyard when my grandmother came by and showed me an injured bird; one of its wings was broken. My grandmother was a nurse and also a shaman, a person who uses natural herbs to cure sickness. As I was watching my grandmother fixing the bird's broken wing, I immediately felt a surge of energy run through me, directing me to help. I knew right then and there what I wanted to be when I grew up. I told my grandmother, "I will become a doctor!" My grandmother agreed, saying that I will become just like her. Therefore, as she raised me, she was imparting her knowledge, beliefs, and techniques to me in how to use herbs to heal.

My mother reinforced my father's and grandmother's words to me, and soon I became a doctor. My father's words echoed in the back of my mind as I studied medicine. I did all the medical protocols I was taught, yet I was always looking for more than what was offered. I wanted to find a different treatment, *the path less traveled to find my answers.* When I told my colleagues, they said, "You are crazy!" But I never quit searching, and with every year, I started to put together treatments that the patients needed to heal.

A significant experience thirty years ago happened when I was working in the ISSTE Hospital; I still remember how my life changed. There was a patient there named Jose. He was sixty-five years old and had prostate cancer with bone, brain, and liver metastases.

One night, as I was listening to his primary doctor, he said to everyone on staff, "The patient in room 35 will be released tomorrow because there is nothing more we can do. We are going to send him home to await his death." At the time this happened, I felt strongly this wasn't right. As doctors, we are not God, and we do not have the power to decide when a person can or cannot die. This experience affected me profoundly, and on that day, I said to myself, *I will work hard and do the best I can with my knowledge, skills, and talents to help patients to cure cancer.*

The next day, as I drove home from the hospital, my mind began to focus; what different approach could I find to start working against the cancer? My father's words echoed in my mind, *Look for the path less traveled to find the answers.*

A series of incidents occurred that made me think, *I will make a cancer vaccine.* Here we have this defense system that Mother Nature gave us in our body; why not use this! So I began to make my first approach for cancer treatment using the immune system of goats to test out my theory. I started to go after cancer by educating the immune system's natural defense system to attack cancer, which is called immunotherapy. This has turned out to be a very effective way to treat cancer.

Money and a partner came along, and soon I became a medical director of my own hospital. For over twenty-five years, I've been privileged to help patients heal cancer, using nontoxic, less invasive methods, including cancer vaccines.

Nearly three decades of research, today I continue to make the vaccines more effective and, year by year, customize the vaccines to be very specific for each cancer cell. I don't use animals for research anymore. I have all the technology I need to perform the vaccines for cancer, like an incubator, a Petri dish, DNA and RNA machines, and genetics to develop the cancer vaccines right from the patient's blood. Chapter 4 will detail all about these immunotherapy protocols.

I remember my first patient in 1987. His name was Dan. His story is in chapter 12. He had a glioblastoma brain tumor, and when we talked, I explained to him about the cancer vaccine, and he said to me, "Dr. Rubio, they gave me only three months to live, let's go and do it." This was over twenty-four years ago, and Dan is living a full and rich life.

As I worked with the immune system and cancer vaccines, I realized I needed to make a protocol like an umbrella to treat cancer. First, I looked at what the cancer cells need to stay alive and move to other organs. Once I understood what the cancer cells need to stay alive, survive, and spread, I began to develop specific therapies for all these conditions to make the immune system educated to attack the invader and strong enough to stop the growth of the cancer cells.

Our expectations come from our beliefs . . .

Our beliefs come from our experiences.

Carolyn Gross's Story

Years ago, while watching a Bill Moyer's special on *Healing and the Mind*, I noticed I was completely fascinated as they showed terminal cancer patients on a weeklong retreat, sharing their lives together. The patients were so authentic in the way they enjoyed this experience at a Santa Barbara retreat center. I wondered why sometimes the real treasures in life don't manifest until we are met with extreme adversity. Never in my wildest dreams did I envision that one day I'd be in a very similar situation.

I always prayed to be an author and motivational speaker. I knew the most important thing for a speaker to be truly great is to have an important message. I was writing my first book, *Staying Calm in the Midst of Chaos*, before the events of September 11, and after the attacks, I realized I have the perfect book for the shift that was occurring in our country.

I began touring my book in 2002, and after eighteen months and twenty-four cities, just when I thought I'd be exhilarated and proud, I felt fatigued and wondered why. This is when I found a lump in my breast and was diagnosed with stage 3 breast cancer, specifically infiltrating ductal carcinoma. The year was 2003, and that ended my book tour.

I went to three doctors: my general practitioner, a surgeon, and an oncologist. All told me the same story—remove the breast immediately! That was the only option given—a complete mastectomy with full courses of chemotherapy and radiation. I couldn't help notice I was being offered the exact same treatment protocols both my grandmothers had received thirty years earlier. I questioned, why haven't we progressed (breast) cancer treatment past the disco era? I was convinced there had to be another option, but I had no clue where or what it was.

It was a desperate couple of weeks for me when I knew I had advanced breast cancer, and I didn't want a mastectomy. I had to find a way out of this precarious position. I started to believe there would be a solution, prayed feverishly, and did a lot of research. I wasn't trying to make history when I went to explore alternative treatment options; I was simply trying to save my breast.

I had many phone calls to trusted friends during desperate days of feelings besieged by impending helplessness and hopelessness. This was a motivational speaker trying to have beliefs and follow her expectations of healing, but it was sheer emotional turmoil. My research introduced me to immunotherapy. At that point, I felt like an airplane that had lost one of the engines and was spiraling down, sure to crash. I heard, through a trusted friend, about a doctor down in Mexico using the immune system to heal cancer. Instantly this reignited my seemingly failing engines. This idea to find a road less traveled to reverse this situation just clicked for me. I went from helpless to hopeful, believing this would be a profound experience.

My natural health and wellness roots served me in making this decision to save my breast with a less invasive cancer treatment protocol. My mother was influenced by her grandmother, a Christian Science practitioner who taught how to use the power of the mind to heal her clients. She always encouraged a nonmedication lifestyle. This led to my interest in natural healing practices, and my father reinforced a special energy I had in my hands when I was very young. I eventually became a massage therapist and had a private practice as a craniosacral therapist. When clients came to me with disc problems and TMJ issues, I'd always suggest, "Make surgery your last resort, it could be a permanent solution to a temporary problem." The idea to start my cancer therapy with cutting off my breast seemed against everything I stood for, especially since the breast didn't cause the cancer! As a woman in her forties with full medical benefits, my husband and I chose to spend our own money to cover my cancer treatment. It was my firm belief that this was the only way to save my life and preserve my health.

Ten years ago, I met Dr. Rubio and had a complete healing of stage 3 breast cancer without *any* surgery, using exclusively his treatment protocols. I spent my early months of cancer treatment documenting this experience and published my second book, *Treatable and Beatable: Healing Cancer without Surgery*—a book that documents the power of the mind, personal healing rituals, and beliefs I used when my own immune system destroyed a 3.5-cm tumor. How many people tell you ten years after a cancer diagnosis, "My immune system is stronger, and I'm healthier after cancer"? This is absolutely my truth.

Today it is my privilege to work as a patient advocate with Dr. Rubio to administer education, encouragement, and hope as part of the team at Rubio Cancer Center. Recently a patient told me, "You have to emphasize that Dr. Rubio's treatment is customized treatment," so here it is—our way to put into your hands the protocols used extensively in *Breaking the Cancer Code*.

Chapter 1

The Fifty-Fifty Relationship

Who do you know that doesn't have their lives touched by cancer? In our own lives, or those of family and friends, cancer is a hot topic today. Within our communities, stories are rampant that demonstrate a need to find a new way out of the cancer predicament.

We truly are at a revolutionary point in breaking the cancer code. Scientists and medical researchers are trying to find multiple ways to successfully heal cancer. The approach discussed in this book will target the most important tool to healing cancer—the patient's own immune system. We will present extensive research done at Rubio Cancer Center with a multitude of successful cancer healings. It is with great joy we bring you this important information. When the idea for this type of noninvasive treatment began, we were one of a handful of cancer centers in the world taking up this approach.

Today, we are delighted that so many scientists and researches are looking to new modalities like immunotherapy, which will be extensively detailed throughout this book. The idea that gene sequencing, epigenetics, and targeted medicines are the forefront of this new approach will all be discussed. We are fortunate for news publications, like the cover of *Time* magazine for April 2013 that read, "How to Cure Cancer*," with a footnote, "*Yes, it's now possible—thanks to new cancer dream teams that are delivering better results faster." The people are ready, and the patients are interested in a new approach.

This material and topic is imperative for a very specific population, and three come to mind immediately:

1. Patients who are diagnosed with cancer and are battling for their lives right now; they are looking to heal and start life over without cancer.
2. People who have been diagnosed with cancer and are healed but suffer with the fear of a recurrence.
3. People who don't have cancer but struggle with *what if?* They live with the idea of getting cancer because it runs in their family.

Whatever group you fit into, we hope you delve into these pages with fervor to help you heal. So many people embark upon the cancer-healing journey, thinking, *If I find the right doctor, everything will be fine.* Others think, *I love my doctor, I'm going to do everything my doctor says and nothing else.* If you can relate to these sentiments, that's great. However, the premise of this book is that this is only half of the equation!

The Healing Partnership

In breaking the cancer code, it's a fifty-fifty relationship. First, there is finding the right doctor and following their advice. However, that is only 50 percent of the equation. Guess what the other essential component of your successful healing is? It's *you*, yes, you, equally weighted with the doctor's orders and efficacy of the medicine. It's your follow-through, your faith, and your effort that make the overall picture complete.

> A patient's positive approach is absolutely essential to ensuring a cancer free life.

Many times people get a diagnosis and think, *It's over*, and they give up. The medicines don't work very well when patients have already resigned themselves to believing that they're through. We've seen this time and time again; a person's "positivity" when diagnosed makes a huge difference. Not only do they overall feel better because of their positive approach, but others feel good around them too, that means doctors, nurses, families, and friends!

Being a Proactive Patient

The proactive patients who take their job of healing seriously seem to succeed. Having worked with thousands of patients over the years, we have clearly observed the successful ones, and success leaves clues. The patients that reverse cancer and successfully heal take 100 percent responsibility for their half of the relationship.

In a funny way, you can compare this to a marriage. Would you go down the aisle and say to your spouse, "My happy marriage is 100 percent in your hands?" If you did, they would probably run! Isn't it more accurate to say to your prospective partner, "This marriage relationship is a partnership, and I'll do my share, you do yours, and we'll likely be happy together."

When you embark upon your healing journey, with your doctor as a partner, you have to be responsible for your half of the relationship. With your doctor providing the medical insights and you as the proactive patient, both doing their share, together you and your doctor will have a successful healing relationship.

This book offers a healing approach that is helpful to breaking the cancer code as discovered and introduced to patients all over the world. We will introduce the expertise of immunotherapy as a methodology that is now accepted more than ever in countries worldwide as a less invasive first-line therapy.

This book actually represents the fifty-fifty approach. Our combined approach from a medical doctor, specializing in using a scientific approach to healing cancer using a powerful weapon, the patient's own immune system! Dr. Rubio at Rubio Cancer Center, with his twenty-eight years of research in immunotherapy and as medical director, will detail how he has helped thousands, and we will outline the treatment he uses throughout this book. We offer a comprehensive protocol, including programs to detoxify and fortify the patient's body.

The other 50 percent of the equation is written by a former stage 3 breast cancer patient, motivational speaker, and health advocate with a voracious appetite for health and healing. Carolyn Gross has been working for nearly a decade with Dr. Rubio as a patient advocate at Rubio Cancer Center. She dedicates herself to educating and empowering patients and their families.

This fifty-fifty relationship does not say that the patient knows as much as the doctor—no way, no how. Doctors are a special breed because they devote themselves to the healing of others and have years upon years of research, study, and application, which cannot be questioned. However, doctors who specialize in cancer often haven't had cancer.

After all their years of studying and helping others, they cannot offer that *inside experience* that only survivors or "thrivers" get a glimpse of. We want to remind patients that you have a special power in your healing, and once you break the cancer code, you have insights that can be applied to every part of your life. Successfully healing cancer gives you a diploma for the rest of your life that says, "I faced death and won." Recently we met a colorectal survivor who told us the title of her book, *If the War Is Over Why Am I Still in Uniform.* Her message is "Cancer gave me a better life!" We like this approach. It's important that once the war is won, you move on with your life.

During a recent lecture to a group of naturopath physicians, we posed this question to this health-educated audience, "What percentage of a patient's getting well is determined by their attitude and mind-set?" The doctors responded 80–90 percent. Please accept that this positive energy is an important power a patient has. It even helps the immune system to make peptides, which activate immunological responses.

We want you to know your power in your healing relationship with your doctors. It has been demonstrated, time and time again, that patients who take their mind and direct it to life no matter what the diagnosis will live longer compared to patients who mentally can't find a way out from under their diagnosis and default to depression or despair.

Diagnosis—the First Step to Healing

When a patient finds a tumor, *bam*, their life shifts immediately! This 180-degree shift happens in every aspect of their being: physically, mentally, emotionally, and spiritually. Normally, confident people can get incapacitated or depressed; normally, calm people can get angry and agitated, and high-strung people tend to get emotional and upset. This reaction is partially physiological, based on the presence of the proteins that do not belong in their body, which the invader cells (cancer) have created. Normal reactions upon diagnosis include shock, self-pity, fright, resentment, mistrust, and a sudden acute awareness of symptoms that were previously ignored.

No matter what the reaction to the diagnosis, in order for patients to heal, they need to find that special combination of medical experts that they can trust to get their critical needs met. From our perspective, the ways to heal cancer successfully include correcting at the cellular level, item by item, the systems of the body that need boosting to support patients to get back their health and, secondly, getting the metabolic system back into balance and homeostasis again.

Getting ready to heal cancer can be a daunting task. Cancer patients have to get educated quickly. Deciding what to do can be the most difficult decision a patient ever makes. There are so many books on the subject because cancer is one of the top diseases. There are many treatment options too, both allopathic (traditional) and alternative.

Proactive Protocol

Proactive patients get engaged immediately to do Internet research so they can see what inclination they want to consider in making their right decision. Listed below are some fifty-fifty patient suggestions:

1. Before going to meet with a medical or health professional, be organized and prepare your questions ahead of time.
2. Let your doctors and medical experts know you are educated and interested so that they see this as they address your specific needs.
3. Interview/investigate what other patients with a similar diagnosis did to heal. Ask the doctor for patient names he's treated.
4. Be open-minded and flexible. If you need to travel and have an extended stay in order to heal, don't let some earthbound (job, kids, or pets) responsibility get in your way.
5. Google your diagnosis, treatment plans, etc. Remember, the Internet may have controversial things to report when you go outside traditional therapies.
6. Investigate! It takes work to get savvy about cancer protocols and treatments, but your life depends upon it.
7. Attend seminars devoted to cancer-specific conferences (e.g., Cancer Control Society, Annie Appleseed Project, Health Freedom Expo, and Your Health is Your Wealth to name a few). For more events, visit www.breakingthecancercode.com. There is a list of resources.
8. To make things convenient, Google health and wellness events in your area.

The Patient Puzzle

To break the cancer code, we will introduce several parts to the patient puzzle of less invasive, natural therapies as a starting point to any cancer-treatment program. We emphasize the starting point here. If we wage a battle against cancer, why would we start with our most aggressive weapon? When you begin a treatment plan with aggressive treatments and the cancer survives, it becomes more aggressive! So if we start treatment *without* the super aggressive drugs and make progress, then the quality of health is spared from being destroyed. You can always strengthen your attack, if needed, in the future. This is why, when treating or advising patients, we initially suggest starting slow and then building the momentum as we go.

As an example of aggressive treatment, a smart patient named Valarie was diagnosed with triple-estrogen-negative breast cancer. She took the full-monty approach to start as her doctors recommended. She had a mastectomy with lymph nodes removed, as well as seven months of chemotherapy and radiation. Her side effects after this treatment were a difficult case of lymphedema, a very painful left side of her body between the tissue extenders of the breast. Four months later, the cancer came back.

In the war on cancer, declared long ago, treatment protocols got very aggressive. Chemotherapies, surgeries, and radiation are still par for the course. Let's just look at chemotherapy for a moment. If a treatment protocol, like Valarie's seven months of chemo, doesn't kill off cancer, guess what can happen? The cancer gets stronger. It's like starting a war with an atomic bomb instead of lobbing a grenade first. In some cases, when patients start off easy to save their body's vitality and remove the cancer, they can rebuild their health with less invasive protocols.

Cancer is a conversation that frequently ends with tough decisions and dismal news. Normally, patients experience fear and powerlessness. The idea that the immune system can fight this condition isn't the consensus. It's hard to have a general consensus when certain medicines aren't FDA approved (yet). Fear and cancer go hand in hand in many traditional treatment sectors. The doctors are the experts that patients rely on for navigation to safe harbors, yet the spiral of fear-infused treatments makes it difficult for many patients to find safe harbors or peace of mind. The premise of this book is to infuse hope into whatever your treatment protocol is. It's time for a change, and as another longtime survivor once said, "God is in the medicine!"

It is our goal to offer hope from experts who specialize in empowering patients with the science developed to teach their immune systems to recognize and reverse cancer, instead of slash, poison, and then burn. Immunotherapy is a treatment approach that empowers patients psychologically while offering a series of integrative treatment protocols to systemically and physically break the cancer code. Once a person has cancer, this is a systematic condition that holds a superior place once activated on a patient's life.

Some cancers are fast growing, wily, and hard to completely destroy. It only takes a few cells to escape the ravages of the "atomic bomb" chemotherapy to start to grow again. When this happens, will the less aggressive therapies work? Our position is to start with the least invasive protocols first, measure the results, and then save the A-bomb for later, if necessary. We get a better result because this way, you won't disrupt homeostasis and healthy cells at the beginning of the battle.

CEO of Your Body

From the bird's-eye view of working at a cancer center, we see firsthand that patients who make it are the ones who know it is *their* job to heal. If nobody has told you before, then listen up. *Patients, you have power. You have the power to heal yourself. Quit giving your power away. Yes, you have a very special power!* As author Chris Carr says in her book titled *Crazy Sexy Cancer*, "You are the CEO or President of your healing." You have at your feet, doctors, experts, and spiritual leaders to assist you, but ultimately, you are in charge of the total operation because you do have the power of choice. In breaking the cancer code, it is important to put some responsibility back into a patient's hand. Your power of yes or no acts like the spoke of a wheel; all facets revolve around the decisions you make.

Sprinkled throughout this book will also be stories of patients' healing with medical strategies that boost the immune system. We want to present several areas where the cancer code begins and how, by addressing each area, we can loosen the grip of cancer and, if you dare, break the cancer code. Before we devote the rest of this book to your healing success and the new technology of immunotherapy, we want to cover the overview of the medical approach.

At Rubio Cancer Center, the protocol of immunotherapy is like an umbrella to treat cancer. First, we look at what the cancer cells need to stay alive and move to other organs. So the cancer cells need

- Nutrition (glucose)
- PH balance
- Anaerobic conditions (no oxygen)
- Angiogenesis (new blood vessels)
- Protein coating
- DNA changes
- Virus like a vector
- Cells that escape from the immune system
- Iron levels
- Stress in platelets
- Hormones: estrogen, testosterone, progesterone

With this understanding of what it takes for the cancer cells to stay alive, survive, and thrive, you will find comprehensive and specific therapies to address all these conditions to break the cancer code and make the immune system strong. This revolutionary approach gives you a strong immune system to live with once you disarm and stop the growth of cancer cells.

Chapter 2

A Brief History of Cancer:
Definition, Causes, and Diagnosis

A Historical Look at What Causes Cancer

Cancer has been around as long as humans have existed and even before. Dinosaur bones, over one hundred million years old, exhibit evidence of cancer. Tissues of well-preserved Egyptian mummies four thousand to five thousand years old have been examined and labeled cancerous.

The Greek physician Hippocrates held that cancer was caused by an imbalance of bodily humors brought on by an improper diet and exercise, as well as differences in climate, age, and season. He believed cancer was an excess of black bile. Second-century physician Galen followed Hippocrates's theories and proposed a strict dietary regimen to treat cancer. His treatments were followed by European and Middle Eastern physicians for some 1,500 years.

A cause-and-effect relationship between the industrial society and cancer causation was first proposed by British surgeon Sir Percival Pott in 1775. He discovered that English chimney sweeps suffered from cancer of the scrotum caused by excessive exposure to chimney soot and tar, and that protective clothing could prevent the occurrence. Marie Curie and her husband, Pierre, who discovered radium, both died of cancer. Unaware of the risks of radiation exposure, both developed the disease, as did their daughter and son-in-law who worked with them.

In the early 1900s, cancer was regarded as such a dreaded disease that doctors considered it unethical to tell a patient the truth or to attempt to treat the condition. Bewildered by its causes, doctors thought cancer was an uncontrollable illness that struck its victims randomly. According to the US census in 1909, cancer was the eighth-leading cause of death, accounting for 4 percent of all deaths that year. Back then, due to lack of early detection and ineffective treatments, anyone who developed cancer ultimately died from it.

A diagnosis of cancer was a virtual death sentence in the early 1900s as well. Very few patients survived. By 1935, only 20 percent of cancer patients lived five years past their diagnosis. It was only when the National Cancer Institute and the American Cancer Society began funding studies in the 1930s and 1940s that the first clues about cancer and more promising treatments began to emerge.

Meanwhile, cancer rates continued to increase in the industrialized world, leading many to believe it is now caused in large part by the myriad of chemicals we are exposed to in our food, air, and water. Pesticides and pollution as well as antibiotics used in the meat and poultry we consume have aggravated homeostasis (the health order and functioning in our bodies) contributing to this illness. Today, we know that cancer occurs naturally in animals and plants. In humans, it has a variety of suspected and known causes, including diet, cigarette smoking, viruses, chemical exposure, and faulty genetics.

Initiators and Promoters of Cancer

Cancer is a disease of cell division, a process known as mitosis, that has gone awry. It typically affects organs where the rate of cell division is the highest. For cancer to develop, a cancer-causing substance (carcinogen) is thought to cause a mutation in a cell's DNA code. As a cell divides and reproduces, this abnormal genetic code is passed on to the new cells, which further divide and reproduce the abnormality, resulting in a cancerous tumor.

Scientists believe cancer is created in a two-step process, with some substances acting as initiators and others acting as promoters of cancerous growth. In the 1940s, Dr. Isaac Berenblum, an Israeli research pathologist, discovered both were required for a cancerous tumor to form. Some substances, such as cigarette smoke, act as both initiators and promoters.

This two-step model for cancer growth explains the sometimes long interval between exposure to carcinogens and cancer's actual development. In the

1950s and '60s, based on laboratory experiments, researchers found a myriad of initiators and promoters, including viruses and genes. Families may pass along faulty DNA codes, thus increasing the cancer risk for offspring. Genetics has gained a role as a cancer initiator.

As there are over one hundred diseases under the cancer banner, it is impossible to generalize about them all. Some cancers spread quickly, others hardly at all. When metastasis occurs, cancer cells can spread to the lymph nodes, bones, liver, and brain.

Scientists suspect that individual susceptibility to disease may play a large role in who gets cancer and who doesn't. Scientists know that the body detects cancer in a small number of cells on a continuous basis and that these clusters are routinely discovered and destroyed by the immune system.

In order for cancer to develop, a cell's DNA code must first be altered by an initiator. Then a promoter causes it to reproduce through mitosis. Because of the protective protein coating most tumors surround themselves with, they then become invisible to the immune system. The tumors flourish instead of being destroyed, and they hog nourishment for themselves, starving off the tissue around them.

As the tumor grows, it cannot interpret the signals sent by normal cells surrounding it, cannot perform its role of mitosis (normal growth of the cells), and forgets the normal rules for cell division. Some cancers spread by killing normal tissue nearby, crushing and stealing nutrients from neighboring cells. Other cancers release enzymes to destroy healthy cells and invade their territory.

Experts now ominously predict that one in three Americans will get cancer at some time in their life. It's the second-leading cause of death in the United States following cardiovascular disease. Cancer, when left untreated, kills the host by robbing the body of nutrients, literally eating away at it, and causing organs and systems to quit functioning.

Contributors to Cancer

In his controversial book *Cancer Wars: How Politics Shapes What We Know and Don't Know about Cancer*, author Robert N. Proctor claims cancer is caused by bad habits, bad working conditions, bad government, and faulty genetics. Chemicals in our air, food, and water are the main culprits.

Cancer most commonly occurs in the skin, lungs, colon and rectum, breast, uterus, and in the blood as leukemia. Since it is a disease of cell division, cancer tends to favor organs where the rates of cell division are highest. Cancer also tends to favor organs most frequently exposed to carcinogenic agents, such as the skin and ultraviolet light from excessive exposure to the sun, the lungs and cigarette smoke, and the large intestine's contact with digestive juices, bile acids, and chemical preservatives from foods.

From the study of diseases in different populations (epidemiology), researchers have associated cancers with certain sets of circumstances. As an example, breast cancer has been associated with women who eat a high-fat diet, have experienced an early onset of menstruation, have a late menopause, and have children late in their lives (after age thirty) or not at all.

Diet and Lifestyle Contributors

Some experts conclude that 76 percent of cancers are caused by lifestyle, including choice of foods, use of tobacco, alcohol consumption, and excessive exposure to the sun.

Some foods and food additives suspected of causing cancer include foods with a high fat content, certain food colorings, nitrites and nitrates used as preservatives, pesticides, and hormone residues in meats. Other contributors are processed fats in foods (i.e., french fries and potato and tortilla chips that make normal cells more susceptible to attack by free radicals floating through the bloodstream).

These things can cause genetic mutations, which potentially develop into cancer. Food preservatives, such as nitrites and nitrates used in lunch meats, convert in the digestive tract into nitrosamines and are proven carcinogens. Hormones and pesticides used to feed chicken and cattle to speed up growth end up as residue in the meats and become carcinogens in our bodies. Excess alcohol has been linked to cancers of the mouth, pharynx, larynx, and esophagus.

An estimated 85 percent of lung cancer is caused by cigarette smoking. Skin cancer is caused mostly by excessive exposure to ultraviolet light from the sun, but genetics and exposure to aromatic hydrocarbons—such as coal tars, soot, asphalt and lubricating oils—can also be factors in its development. Cancers of the skin and leukemia often develop from overexposure to radiation and x-rays as well. Pollutants and workplace carcinogens—including asbestos, benzene, and polyvinyl chloride—can lead to the development of cancer twenty to thirty years after exposure.

Causes of Abnormal Cell Growth

As discussed, normal cells grow with a control mechanism for cell division that we call mitosis. When a tumor develops at the cellular level, cancer cells grow without any control. In the normal process of mitosis, a cell undergoes a metabolic reaction that requires specific amino acids to build blocks of proteins to replicate chromosomes and produce an identical cell.

At the cellular level of the patient who develops a tumor, one of two amino acids is deficient: either glutamine or arginine. When either of these amino acids is not present to build a new protein, the cell loses control, causing an abhorrent chemical reaction to take place, and a cancerous cell can grow. Carcinogens cause cancer to appear as abhorrent RNA and DNA fragments, and viruses take the place of missing normal amino acids during mitosis, producing an abnormal cell.

Food can be one cause of loading the cells with carcinogenic chemicals. On the cellular level, these chemicals adversely affect the cell and its DNA and can produce or accelerate the appearance of a tumor. Pesticides, preservatives, radiation, and unfiltered water laden with a lot of added chemicals, such as chlorides and fluorides, all put pressure on the normal cell environment.

Researchers have also found that missing chromosomes, principally chromosome 3, are the first causes of cancers in cells of the breasts, lungs, brain, liver, stomach, and colon. In these types of cancer, the absence of chromosome 3 allows a virus to invade normal cells, attach themselves where chromosome 3 should be, and use the organ to grow quickly and replicate. This leads to a process that develops into a tumor within five to eight years.

The defective proteins in the cancer cells protect themselves with a protein coating that prevents the immune system from detecting and destroying them. The proteins create what we call blocking factors. Additionally, the cells are in constant change and disguise themselves as normal cells, causing the immune system to fail to recognize them. With cancer, the immune system is unable to destroy these abhorrent proteins or to penetrate the protective protein coating around tumors. These proteins also change their coating to camouflage themselves and escape detection from the immune system.

PH Levels: Amino Acids

Cancer cells are simple cells. They don't require a complex metabolic reaction to grow. Cancer cells grow from fermentation. The pH level around the cells is very acidic. This anaerobic environment makes the tumor grow quickly. It is difficult to direct the immune system to attack the cancer because the environment prevents amino acids and oxygen from getting through.

Doctors who focus on multiple therapies that work to reverse cancer cells to create healthy cells are finding greater success. The research of our medical team uses specific amino acids for specific chemical reactions, where the amino acids glutamine and arginine cause the missing chromosomes to reappear and stop the process of the cancer's growth.

Dr. Rubio's immunotherapy research team has been committed to breaking the cancer code, using therapies that have been focused on programming the immune system to recognize and destroy the errant cancer cells.

How Doctors Diagnose and Classify Cancers

Cancer patients don't know they have a tumor until they have symptoms. The tumor will impinge on nerves, causing pain, or a big mass will be detected in the body. Most tumors need five to ten years to develop, starting out very small on the cellular level. However, some tumors grow very fast and can multiply in size within weeks or days. This happens in certain melanoma, lung, brain, and ovarian cancers.

Listed below are general symptoms that indicate a patient should see a physician immediately. Different types of cancer have different symptoms, so if you are only experiencing a couple of warning signs, it's best to check with your doctor.

Cancer symptoms include the following:

- Night fevers
- Night sweats
- Progressive weight loss
- Bleeding from the rectum or stomach
- Repetitious infections
- A mass in a breast
- A breast discharge or an inverted nipple
- Hard lymph nodes in the neck or under the arms

- Excessive bruising
- Coughs with blood
- Pain in the bones
- Headaches
- Nausea or vomiting
- Blood in the saliva
- Inflammation in the testicles
- Itching
- Pain in the hips or spine
- Skin ulcers
- Moles changing form or color
- Difficulty eating, swallowing, or breathing
- Trouble urinating
- Difficulty with bowel movements
- Bleeding from the vagina

Here are some methods for early determination before cancer appears. Cancer can be diagnosed by examining genetics, as well as family origins, and checking for chromosome 3. With a specific test for breast cancer, BRCA1 and BRCA2 determine family genetics.

The five steps of cancer development include the following:

1) Amino acid deficiency allows abhorrent mitosis.
2) Blocking factors protect growth of tumor.
3) Escape of immune detection prevents destruction.
4) Anaerobic environment enhances cancer growth.
5) pH/acid balance disruption affects normal metabolism.

The AMASS is an antibody test that can show cancer cells before a tumor shows up. This new blood test called the AMASS test will look for specific antibodies and tumor markers, both signs of cancer before the tumor shows up. After a physical examination, the doctor may utilize a series of tools and diagnostic exams to determine if cancer is present. From an x-ray, CAT scan, and magnetic resonance imaging (MRI), the doctor may notice a mass or tumor in a different organ from the original complaint. Ultrasound and mammograms may also detect tumors.

With a biopsy (the surgical removal of a small portion of the mass), the doctor will obtain a conclusive final diagnosis of cancer. When a tumor is cut into, the cancer is going to escape the tumor and spread. It is necessary for doctors to confirm a diagnosis within two days so they can quickly administer techniques for stopping the tumor from spreading. The traditional uses of chemotherapy, radiation, and surgery will stop the tumor from spreading.

Types of Cancer

Below is a list of the types of cancer that are named by region.

- Adrenal
- Anus
- Bile duct
- Bladder
- Breast
- Cancer of an unknown primary site
- Carcinoids of the gastrointestinal tract
- Cervix
- Childhood cancers
- Colon and rectum
- Esophagus
- Gallbladder
- Head and neck
- Islet cell and other pancreatic carcinomas
- Kaposi's sarcoma
- Kidney
- Leukemia
- Liver
- Lung: non-small cell
- Lung: small cell
- Lymphoma: AIDS associated
- Lymphoma: Hodgkin's disease
- Lymphoma: non-Hodgkin's
- Melanoma
- Mesothelioma
- Metastatic cancer
- Multiple myeloma
- Ovary
- Ovarian germ cell tumors
- Pancreas
- Parathyroid
- Penis
- Pituitary
- Prostrate
- Sarcomas of bone and soft tissue

- Skin
- Small intestine
- Stomach
- Squamous Cell
- Testis
- Thymus
- Thyroid
- Trophoblastic disease
- Uterus: endometrial carcinoma
- Uterus: uterine sarcomas
- Vagina and vulva

TNM System of Staging

The TNM system of staging has been developed to provide a similar classification system for tumors worldwide. The letter T refers to the size of the tumor; N indicates the rate of spread to the lymph glands, and M describes the level of metastasis throughout the body. Numbers following each letter, from 0 to 4, tell the size and spread of the tumor.

As an example, T 0 indicates a tumor was completely removed by biopsy. T 1 through T 4 relates to various sizes of tumors, with T 4 being the largest. A classification of N 0 means there was no spread of the cancer to lymph nodes. N 1 through N 4 indicates increasing presence of cancer in the lymph system. M 0 indicates no distant metastasis; M 1 indicates distant metastasis.

A TNM classification with lower numbers greatly increases the chances of a complete remission; a TNM classification with higher numbers indicates an advanced stage of cancer that may be more difficult to cure. By standardizing the TNM system for doctors and cancer researchers around the world, the efficacy of various treatments can be measured with a common criterion.

Taking the TNM numbers into account, doctors' group cancer in stages I through stage IV, with stage IV being the most serious and metastasized. Once the tumor is categorized in such a way, doctors can develop a specific treatment protocol that has shown the best results in previous cases.

Trending Toward the Future

Now that we've covered the past and are looking at the twenty-first century forward, cancer patients have a 50 percent chance of recovery using only traditional medicine. The success rate is higher in a few cancers, such as non-Hodgkin's lymphoma and testicular cancer.

What we have found in extensive work with cancer patients, which will be reported in the next several chapters, is that doctors using both traditional medical treatments and nontraditional protocols have the greatest success in reversing cancer.

This continued interest and emphasis will allow more natural solutions to cross over into cancer treatment. Research is now continuous in the cancer field within hospitals and universities across the country, combining natural therapies with pharmaceutical solutions. We see this global trend happening now, and the results are promising!

Just as many American doctors today are recognizing the value of diet and nutritional substances in preventing and aiding in healing many diseases, we know this is a hopeful sign that patients will realize personal responsibility (the fifty-fifty relationship) and the lifestyle change needed for successful healing.

Chapter 3

Immunotherapy:
Advancing Cancer Treatment

> Many of the truths we cling to depend upon . . .
> our own point of view.

Immunotherapy is one of the newest and most advanced types of therapies available to treat cancer. It is also one of the hottest areas of research in the United States, with many promising studies showing positive results in treating disease conditions, both in humans and animals. Immunotherapy enhances the body's unique ability to heal itself from the inside out, instead of therapies that work from the outside in, such as surgery.

Another feature story in *Time* magazine years ago featured an issue on the war against cancer, announcing immunotherapy as one of the treatment options to hit the scoreboard in cancer treatment. Research testing vaccines for cancer has been underway in the United States for years as a primary and adjunct treatment protocol. The FDA has currently approved some cancer vaccines for prostate cancer and the human papillomavirus, which can be a precursor to ovarian cancers.

Cancer Vaccines: A Primary Treatment

Every day, more doctors and biologists are recognizing through research that immunotherapy is a viable treatment option. We are thrilled to be part of the forefront of this research in breaking the cancer code! Our medical team of chemist and doctors have developed a series of remarkable vaccines from components of a patient's own body and cancer cells. We discovered this treatment can impart information to the natural defenses of the patient's body to effectively stop and destroy cancerous tumors. This approach forms the heart of extensive research and our time-tested, unique treatment program at Rubio Cancer Center. This book is the beginning of our way to share this exciting information with you, as many cancer centers around the world are adding cancer vaccines to their treatment lineups. We will be offering educational seminars on this. For further information, visit www. breakingthecancercode.com

Using the Immune System to Heal Cancer

When properly awakened, a patient's immune system already has all the tools necessary to detect, attack, and destroy cancer. The only way to completely stop cancer is through enhancing the function of the immune system. Since this has been the cornerstone of the unique therapies, we advocate these therapies to help fortify the patient's internal systems to make their own immune system stronger. This is vitally important for cancer patients during and after treatment.

To achieve this goal, immunotherapy protocols, developed over twenty-eight years, have been proven; from breast cancer to colon cancer and brain tumors to lung cancer—all have been reversed successfully. There have been hundreds of successes with advanced stage and rare cancers like mesothelioma or embryonic, W germ cell cancers as well as more common ones. Our research found the vaccines to be especially effective when used in conjunction with low doses of chemotherapy and radiation. People seeking natural methods get dismayed when they hear of this, but the dose we recommend is not intended to destroy the cancer but to contain it from spreading as well as weaken it. The primary method of destroying cancer is left to the immune system.

Our Immune System at a Glance

Our immune system is the defense mechanism that protects us against negative influences, such as antigens, proteins, bacteria, chemicals, and cancerous cells that can cause us to become sick or develop diseases. It is composed of various types of white blood cells called lymphocytes, whose numbers increase in response to infections and diseases, including cancer.

There are two primary types of immunity in the body: Humoral, composed of B cells, which produce antibodies that attack foreign cells and the cellular, composed of T cells, which react to and attack specific foreign substances or viruses. Both components are formed principally in the bone marrow, with the T cells maturing in the thymus.

Killer T cells attach themselves to specific foreign cells and secrete substances to destroy the invaders. They make up about 25 percent of all T cells in the body. Helper T cells secrete interleukins, interferon, and other immune proteins to stimulate B cells and killer T cells to attack foreign invaders. About 65 percent of all T cells are helper T cells. Another T cell called the suppressor T cells turn off excessive reactions by the immune system and suppresses activity of the antibodies.

There is also another important type of white blood cells called the natural killer (NK) cells. They are neither B nor T cells and are equipped with an arsenal of up to one hundred different poisons to quickly recognize and kill foreign invaders. All these components of the immune system work to survey the inner systems of the body and quickly scour it of foreign cells and antigens (i.e., strange proteins).

Immunotherapy Educates and Targets the Immune System

The immune system is empowered to stop any illnesses in the body. But with patients who have developed cancer, there has been a breakdown, and the immune system does not recognize the cancer as an abnormal growth. Through utilizing the immunotherapy protocols to break the cancer code, our overall goal is to educate and empower the immune system to go to the tumor and recognize, destroy, and eliminate it from the body.

As part of our extensive research, an important first step is to destroy the camouflage protein coating of the cancer cell. This is done by utilizing enzymes to break the protective protein coating. The enzymes essentially implode the coating, making small holes in it.

Getting Rid of Cancer's Blocking Factor

As stated earlier, the reason why the body's natural defense mechanisms are unable to recognize a cancerous tumor is because it hides behind a specific camouflage, a protein coating that acts as a blocking factor. The immune system does not recognize the protein as foreign because this camouflage (blocking factor) masks itself to look like the organ it is attached to. As the immune system (T and NK cells) patrol the body, it passes by as if the cancer is a normal protein and does not attack the cancer. To the immune system, it's as if no problem cells exist at all. This demonstrates how effective the blocking factor is at keeping cancer alive.

From years of laboratory testing, the best method for breaking away the protein coating is by utilizing specific protolytic enzymes and amino acids with specific carriers. In this way, you expose the cells, which is like putting targets on the tumors, and this creates a pathway for the immune system to attack the invader cancer cells. With this approach, the cancer cells form a receptor and send a signal to the immune system. When the vaccine is administered, the educated T cells can attack and know where to go to destroy the tumor.

Sometimes, the tumor escapes detection and destruction by the immune system because the cancer cells change the protein coating of the camouflage. When this happens, the immune system does not have the intelligence to recognize the new camouflage, and once again, the tumor starts to grow.

Cancer Camouflage and Recurrence

Take as an example a primary tumor manifesting as adenocarcinoma in the breast. Traditional methods of treatment include chemotherapy, radiation, surgery, and hormone therapy. After six months in remission, the cancer shows up again, metastasized to the bones, liver, lungs, or brain. Why does this occur?

We know cancer cells are wily invaders by the way they attempt to preserve their existence once they start to grow. Cancer cells are intelligent and will do anything to stay alive. During the exposure to chemotherapy and radiation, cancer cells may be arrested and quit growing and dividing, but as is often the case, not all the cancer cells will be killed. They will hide away in different glands and wait until the effects of chemotherapy and radiation diminish. When the coast is clear, they will then grow back with a different camouflage that is resistant to the chemotherapy they were treated with. They have transformed themselves as a survival mechanism.

For over twenty-five years, through trial and error, Dr. Rubio's medical team simultaneously administers the vaccines along with low doses of chemotherapy and radiation. In this way, we wipe out the tumor so it has less of a chance to change, form, and return. We peel away the protective protein coating, exposing the tumor, which allows the immune system to intelligently attack it. We use a variety of various vaccines to keep the immune system updated and informed. There's a 60–80 percent rate to reverse the cancer at this point. These odds are generally better than what would be expected with traditional methods alone.

Immunotherapy Combined with Chemotherapy and Radiation

Chemotherapy and radiation offer substantial benefits to the cancer patient. (More information is detailed in chapter 4). They allow an enhanced immune system to work against fewer cancer cells and give it greater odds to destroy the cancer. With cancer, the immune system is overwhelmed, with one fighter cell against twenty-five cancer cells. The immune system has little chance of winning; sooner or later the cancer will kill the host.

Through immune-enhancing therapies, like the cancer vaccines, we increase the number of immune system cells from five billion to perhaps seven billion cells. At the same time, the low doses of chemotherapy and radiation may reduce the number of cancer cells from twenty-five billion to ten billion. By leveling the playing field, the odds are more even, which gives patients a much better chance of conquering cancer.

After years of tests and trials, our medical team's research has come up with five different types of vaccines to train the immune system to attack and destroy the cancer. They are named as follows: passive vaccine, active vaccine, nonspecific vaccine, specific vaccine, and dendritic vaccine. The rest of this chapter will detail the characteristics of each vaccine.

Passive Vaccine

The passive vaccine was developed to facilitate a process we call RNA transference to the lymphocytes. In this RNA transference, one white blood cell transmits information to other white blood cells to attack the cancer.

The procedure for making the vaccine begins when we obtain a piece of the tumor from the patient's own body. We perform either a needle biopsy or surgical biopsy to extract a piece of the tumor. The next step is to culture these cancer cells in the laboratory. In those cases where surgery is too risky to obtain a piece of the tumor, we use the patient's own blood, urine, or spinal fluid as a substitute. There are tumor markers in these fluids called antigens, which can be very useful to create the vaccine as well.

So with two different blood samples, one extracted for the cancer cells, we withdraw another. This one is for white blood cells we extract from the patient's blood as well. We add these white blood cells to the cancer culture with specific carriers, and the white blood cells then attack the cancer cells and destroy them.

By doing this, these white blood cells will gain a specific memory of the shape and type of genes of the tumor. This memory now gives them the method and power to destroy the tumor in the future. The white blood cells now can recognize the RNA code of the cancer and its particular proteins.

The process for creating RNA transference of the lymphocytes takes twenty-one days in the laboratory. These white blood cells now have the memory and ability to recognize the tumor and attack it. Taking the educated white blood cells from the culture, we inject them back into the patient's bloodstream.

Preparing for the Vaccine

By this time, specific washing factors and protocols have already been employed to penetrate the cancer's protective protein coat. The educated white blood cells, which have memorized the cancer's protein makeup, are attracted to the exposed tumor. They are programmed to attack and destroy it, as well as any similar metastasized cancer cells.

An important benefit of the vaccine is that the educated T cells will send messages to the bone marrow of the patient and direct it to produce copies of the same type of T cells that are programmed to attack the cancer. When a patient has a very large established tumor, it is difficult for the immune system to destroy it completely. In these situations, one T cell may be pitted against ten or even one hundred opponents. Obviously, in this instance, the immune system doesn't have a good chance of winning.

By using intelligent therapies first to remove or diminish the number of cancer cells, this allows an opportunity for the immune system to work one-on-one or ten-to-one against the cancer. As discussed earlier, we use a low dose of radiation and chemotherapy to diminish the amount of cancer cells and stop their growth first, giving the immune system the advantage and changing the odds toward victory.

Because the passive vaccine is created from proteins extracted from one's own body, patients don't experience as many devastating side effects from the vaccine as they do from traditional chemotherapy and radiation treatments. They may have fever, muscle aches, and headaches for twenty-four to forty-eight hours following the injection. However, these symptoms are not side effects; they are symptoms that occur because a lot of activities are taking place internally. We call these symptoms pyrogen endogenous, meaning to increase or raise the temperature.

Once the Cancer Is Destroyed, Where Does It Go?

While the vaccine is working, the white blood cells are attacking the tumor, and the tumor is starting to die. What happens when the tumor dies, and where does it go? The tumor liquefies or breaks into pieces; the protein fragments enter the bloodstream and are processed through the lymph system.

The lymphatic system begins to overload with waste as T cells with encapsulated pieces of the tumor are processed through the lymph system and redeposited in the bloodstream. The dead tumor cells, protein poisoning, and other wastes from the process are then eliminated through the kidneys, liver, colon, and skin. Doctors and patients need to be aware that when using this method to destroy tumors, we are creating protein poisons and free radicals. It's important to detoxify these organs of elimination in advance to allow them to function optimally to drain the wastes of cancer destruction from the body.

Within three to five weeks, we often see a reduction in the tumor's size following the use of the vaccine, as well as the intensity of any accompanying pain diminishing. The effects of the passive vaccine last up to three months. After three months, the RNA transference of the white blood cells starts to decline, and the vaccine has to be repeated. As the number of T-cells diminishes, more cancer cells escape from the immune system, changes their protein makeup, and don't receive the beneficial effects of the vaccine.

We have to repeat the process because cancer adapts quickly and becomes resistant as it transforms itself while fighting for its survival. To survive, the cancer will change its protein coating, and its cells will change.

To continue with the healing process,
we need to keep the immune system continuously informed and updated.

Customized Cancer Care

Traditional methods—such as the use of antibodies, interleukin-2 through interleukin-13, and interferon—are good for awakening the immune system to try to destroy the tumor, but genetic differences among patients will affect results. In general, on its own, interleukin is not completely effective against individual cancers. The problem with some of the traditional methods is that they don't work for everyone because of different genetic makeup's.

We are now seeing that cancer requires us to work individually with each patient, and this method of customized care is how we'll break the cancer code and advance cancer treatment. Each patient has an individual map for healing and recovery; we need to discover this map or code to make the therapy programs work physically, mentally, and emotionally. Following a generalized map in medicine sometimes ignores individual differences.

At Rubio Cancer Center, our team works out an individual program of patient care. We know from experience that a successful individual program recognizes the constant changes taking place internally, with everything moving and changing metabolically in the cancer-healing process. Our body is alive, constantly changing. Therefore, we suggest treating cancer with live therapies, such as the vaccines.

The passive vaccine works to eradicate any type of cancer in the body. The use of this vaccine is a key to the effectiveness of our successful programs. Chemotherapy and radiation may shrink and stop the tumor for a while but will not destroy it completely. This vaccine works to destroy cancer completely. In using the passive vaccine, combined with low doses of radiation and low doses of chemotherapy, we've witnessed hundreds of advanced-stage patients exhibit remarkable results.

Lymphomas

In 135 cases of applying the passive vaccine to patients with non-Hodgkin's, T cells, B cells, Hodgkin's, and mantle cell lymphoma, we have seen a dramatic reduction of up to 60 percent in tumors of the lymph nodes. Using the passive vaccine against lung cancer, a type of adenocarcinoma, we have caused the tumor to become encapsulated and stop growing. In three months, we've observed the reduction of the tumor.

Lung

In over seventy-five lung cancer patients, the tumors have decreased in size, and in over forty patients, we'd seen the tumors shrink completely. See chapter 10 for a variety of patient success stories.

Liver Cancer

In forty-five patients with liver cancer, we've injected a low dose of chemotherapy directly into the artery leading into the liver. This combined with a nontoxic medication, carbomide, along with the passive vaccine and interferon has been very successful at reversing cancer. We've witnessed a dramatic change in the size of the tumor after it has been put under control, this confirmed by CAT scans. Spots in the pancreas and the liver then start to decrease in density, and the liver begins functioning normally again.

In these forty-five cases, we have never had any complication into the occlusion (plug) in the main duct that drains from the liver and the pancreas. Only in two cases did we have to put a stent in to drain the bile from the liver and the enzymes from the pancreas.

A Way to Stop the Pain

After the application of the passive vaccine to patients with metastasized bone cancer, we've observed greatly diminished pain, so much so that we've been able to stop administering all narcotics and painkillers. This step proves vital for patients to fully recover. Painkillers not only diminish pain, but they block vitality in the body and halt detoxification and elimination cycles in the body. We use lipids of amino acids and specific enzymes that are able to increase endorphins and immediately reduce the pain.

Because of the versatility of success in working with the passive vaccine, our research shows that it is one of the most effective of all our specific cancer therapies.

Nonspecific Vaccine

The efficacy of all the vaccines starts with the nonspecific vaccine. This is where immunotherapy starts to activate the immune system. Since the advent of medicine, doctors have attempted to work intelligently to stop illnesses by using tools that enhance the body's innate healing abilities. Through this research, they have found that using different compounds can awaken or stimulate the immune system. In the use of nonspecific vaccines, as the name implies, we stimulate the immune system in a general way to increase the number of white cells and stimulate their attraction to attack a specific target.

We create nonspecific vaccines through combining different types of lipids from bacteria. These lipids are strong immune boosters. We've been working with nonspecific vaccines created with lipids from activated BCG/tetanus, a combination of BCG (Bacillus Calmette-Guérin) and tetanus.

To administer the vaccine, we inject different types of bacteria *in a non-active state* under the skin. We've seen these lipids grow similarly to the way the cancer grows. When we apply the deactivated bacteria, the capsule of lipids grows in competition with the tumor, both for space and nourishment, and helps to starve the tumor.

The lipids around these bacteria also stimulate the immune system to increase the production of white blood cells. The strengthened immune system can then take advantage of the tumor in its weakening state and start working to eradicate it. This sets the stage for the RNA transference process three weeks later with the passive vaccine. The process is similar to tuning up the engine of a racing car before the race.

BCG and Nonspecific Vaccines

Both BCG (Bacillus Calmette-Guérin) and nonspecific vaccines can also be used, like insurance, to prevent the development of cancer. In countries such as Mexico and South America, children are vaccinated with the BCG vaccine when they are born. The incidence of cancer is much lower. It seems the BCG vaccine greatly protects the human body from developing tumors later in life. BCG vaccines have been in existence since the 1840s when they were developed against tuberculosis. Currently, these vaccines are beginning to be researched again, after years of falling out of use in the United States.

As a therapy, nonspecific vaccines are applied under the skin every week or two. The patient may develop fever, runny nose, muscle aches, rash or a pimple in reaction to application of BCG. Patients need not fear this vaccination; as we have stated, the BCG is not in an active state, rather containing only the lipids that we've extracted from the BCG.

Melanoma

Research in clinical practice has shown that application of BCG as an immunotherapy is effective for melanomas, acute lymphoblast leukemia (ALL and AML), lymphomas, and skin cancer. The nonspecific vaccines have proven to be effective against ALL and AML when used in conjunction with low doses of chemotherapy (vincristine) and specific hormone blockers. High doses of chemotherapy are unnecessary; through these therapies alone, we have been successful in putting the bone marrow into complete remission.

Breast Cancer

In using the nonspecific vaccines with breast cancer, combined with hormone blockers, we've witnessed a rapid reduction in the tumor's size. Nonspecific vaccines are applied as part of the treatment during the first week of therapy and following completion of the first segment of the diet and nutritional program. Nonspecific vaccines are an immune system booster that sets the stage to support the passive vaccine in the weeks that follow.

Active Vaccines

Active vaccines are a wonderful and amazing technique to activate and direct the immune system against tumors. For a long time, doctors have worked with these types of vaccines and witnessed remarkable responses. Our method of customization makes these vaccines unique and tailor-made for each individual patient to activate and educate their own immune system.

To formulate the active vaccine, we obtain a piece of the tumor from the patient through surgery or a needle biopsy to get the cancer cells. When we cannot obtain cancer cells, we use antigens from the blood or urine to make the vaccine. Then we remove the protein coating from the extracted tumor cells and apply a low dose of radiation to slow down or kill them. At the same time, we are careful to not destroy the DNA or genes of the cancer cells. Next we add specific lipids and polypeptides to the dead cancer cells and inject this combined substance back into the patient, under the skin and intramuscularly.

Immediately this preparation produces a big reaction in the patient's body as T cells and the horde of white cells rush to the site of the inoculation and begin to attack and destroy the foreign proteins, lipids, and polypeptides.

This activation against these foreign-looking proteins and lipids stimulates the immune system to recognize the tumor itself as a foreign body and to begin to attack and destroy it as well.

A huge advantage in the active vaccine is that it also stimulates bone marrows to produce and send even more T cells to attack the foreign proteins and lipids. While attacking these strange proteins, the activated immune system will also attack the proteins of the cancer and will search throughout the body for the foreign proteins as metastasized cancer cells can be found in the liver, brain, lymph glands, etc.

Typically, our team uses active vaccines during the second week of therapy in conjunction with interferon and interleukin-12. The cancers that respond most effectively are solid tumors (i.e., adenocarcinomas, melanomas, sarcomas, and cancers of the breast, stomach, lungs, and colon). It prevents tumor growth by blocking the formation of new blood vessels to nourish the tumor. Dramatic changes reducing the tumor size take place following the use of these therapies.

As with the other immunity boosters, the active vaccine works well in advance to support the strongest vaccine, which follows at the end of the third week, the passive vaccine. With these types of vaccines and immunological therapies, the immune system gets stronger, more alert, and harder working, giving the patient an opportunity for the cancer to be destroyed.

The active vaccine, in use for the past twenty-eight years, has been very successful, working specifically with melanomas. We've seen patients with melanomas that have spread to the bones, liver, blood, and brain respond to the active, passive, and nonspecific vaccines combined with interferon. The pain diminishes, and the tumors stop growing. With fibril carcinomas, lymphosarcomas, and leiomyosarcomas, we see dramatic changes in tumor size and the tumor arrested. The active vaccine works synergistically with all the other therapies—including chemotherapy, radiation, herbs, and natural methods—to powerfully deal with the cancer.

Specific Vaccines

For the past sixty years, doctors, biologists, and chemists have tried to find ways to stop cancer, and they started experimenting using different types of bacteria to awaken the immune response. The specific vaccines work by using bacteria to put pressure on the tumor and compete for food and territory. To make the vaccine, we can use active staphylococci, pneumococci, or *Clostridium tetani*. We need to remember that our bodies already function as a big culture for many kinds of fungi and viruses, and we can use this environment to our advantage to help stop the tumor in some cases.

Breast Cancer Study

In a significant study back in 1940 involving forty patients, Dr. Rote applied a staph infection as a last resort to patients with metastasized breast cancer who had already undergone a mastectomy (removal of the breast) and lymphadenectomy (removal of the lymph glands). The patients were experiencing tremendous edema (swelling) and had tumors in their arms. The patients' tumors had spread, and they no longer had a functioning lymphatic system and were considered terminal.

Other efforts to stop the swelling had failed. Dr. Rote intentionally incubated a staph infection on the patients' arms by cutting or scratching them and introducing the infection. He allowed the symptoms of a staph infection to develop. Dr. Rote waited ten days and then used antibiotics to stop the staphylococci. Out of forty patients, twenty patients died from the staph infection, ten did not respond, but for ten patients, not only did the swelling diminish, but the tumors disappeared.

We are not advocating this technique as the preferred solution, but it can be used when other options have failed. These types of therapies are risky, of course. They are only employed when the patient doesn't have any other chance to recuperate and the pressure cannot be relieved in any other way.

Specific vaccines need to be applied carefully in difficult situations and in specific cases. They are especially effective when it is difficult to reverse a large tumor or edema that does not respond to other therapies. We have different bacteria that we can use in the inoculations, such as active staphylococci, pneumoccoci, or *Clostridium tetani*. The specific vaccines can be used daily or weekly in a safe way to stimulate the immune system to create more white cells and alert the patient's body for the next series of vaccines.

The Immune System Is the Key

A missing link we hope to bring to cancer treatments today is using the immune system. The immune system is the key that unlocks the door to successful recovery from cancer. In earlier years, chemotherapies were destroying this system, but improvements have happened in the last several decades to make chemotherapy more user-friendly. We hope people will learn more about how precious and powerful the immune system is to protect them in all conditions, including cancer.

Chapter 4

Radiation and Chemotherapy

The words *radiation* and *chemotherapy* strike up fear and dread in the minds of most cancer patients. They naturally conjure up images of devastating side effects associated with these protocols. Consequently, when a cancer patient's doctor recommends chemotherapy or radiation, we suggest the patient get at least one or two different opinions before consenting to these therapies.

However, radiation and chemotherapy can be beneficial when combined properly. Some cancer tumors—such as lymphomas, leukemia, squamous cell, and oat cell—do respond and begin to shrink. Some chemotherapy and radiation are also used when patients are in extreme pain to prevent paralysis if the tumor is impinging on nerves and also in cases of bone metastasis to prevent fractures from bones weakened by fast-growing cancer cells.

Radiation Backstory

Radiation was developed during the early 1900s through the work of German professor of physics Wilhelm Conrad Roentgen, who discovered x-rays, and Marie and Pierre Curie, who discovered radium in Paris in 1903. It was observed that x-rays and radium caused damage to body tissues. Shortly thereafter, x-rays were used to combat cancer.

The electromagnetic radiation used today is a combination of x-rays (electrically produced) and gamma radiation from the decay of radioactive isotopes. Different ranges and levels of intensity are used on patients.

45

Scientists know radiation damages DNA, and in large-enough dosages, it kills cells. The goal of radiation therapy is always to kill cancer cells while reducing damage to accompanying normal tissues.

Cancer cells are usually more sensitive to radiation than adjacent normal cells. Radiation works in types of cancer cells, such as squamous cell, lung tumors, oat cell, and small cell. We also can apply the radiation to other types of cancers to make the tumors shrink and give an opportunity for the immune system to deal with a decreased number of tumor cells. Side effects may include fatigue, skin changes, hair loss, nausea, and vomiting.

Protocols to Detoxify Radiation

For those going through radiation and chemotherapy, here is another method to maximize the benefits and minimize the side effects. For example, the standard treatment protocol for bone cancer is to use 5,000 rads of radiation. However, in the approach we've been talking about, we use only 500 rads. That is correct, one-tenth of the normal dosage. However, we are using a comprehensive protocol with not only the cancer vaccines, but we also detoxify the body immediately after each radiation treatment by using specific techniques, such as green cabbage poultices, to remove radiation and chemotherapy from the metabolic system. People roll their eyes at first when we tell them about the green cabbage poultices, but the reason they are effective is because of an enzyme, alpha glycerol (from green cabbage), that protects the patient's healthy red and white blood cells from radiation damage and helps to remove radiation from the body. This is our first step in detoxification specifically from radiation.

We also recommend patients use balneotherapy (bath therapy) in which we have our patients take a detox bath before going to bed every night. We use a mixture of baking soda, sea salt, and ginger added to hot bathwater to remove radiation from the body.

Here is how we use the skin to detoxify the side effects of radiation. We ask patients to soak for twenty minutes in a bath of hot water, as hot as possible, since the sweating from this bath is how the toxins exit the body. Next, patients take a tepid shower to rinse the toxins off the skin. This is a very simple yet effective bath for many reasons. The ginger stimulates the body for a bit more energy, and the sea salt remineralizes the patient.

Dead Sea Salt Recipe

Mix ¾ cup Dead Sea salts, 3 tbsp. ginger (powdered ginger), and 1 tbsp. baking soda. Put all ingredients into bath. If Dead Sea salts aren't available, use Epsom salts or mineral salts.

In treating our patients, we want to eliminate radiation from the bloodstream. We do achieve this by using an intravenous infusion of EDTA chelation. EDTA is an approved method in nuclear medicine to remove chemotherapy and radiation from the system. It also removes heavy metals, plaque, and chemicals from the bloodstream. At the same time we use radiation, we allow the patient to breathe oxygen. This enhances the action of the radiation on the tumor.

Kinder and Gentler Chemotherapy and Radiation

Many people interested in natural health are resistant to both chemotherapy and radiation. However, with advanced cancer especially, we have to accept radiation therapy as an approach to help destroy the cancer. From a doctor's perspective, we suggest that medical professionals explain to their patients very honestly the effects. Specifically that through the use of radiation, they are going to destroy a lot of proteins. The dead proteins will be floating in the patient's bloodstream and could create additional problems unless they are quickly removed. That's why in breaking the cancer code, detoxification programs are so important in reversing cancer by supporting the patient to eliminate dead cancer cells and proteins.

We like to think of this as a kinder, gentler, and more specific version of chemotherapy and radiation because patients often do not lose their hair or experience burns to the skin. We want radiation and chemotherapy protocols combined with immunotherapy and metabolic programs to soften or eliminate most of the negative side effects of the traditional, standard cancer treatments.

The goal, as stated earlier, in using radiation or chemotherapy is to destroy millions of cancer cells and to not deplete the patient's immune system in the process. With these innovative methods, we provide the immune system with the information it needs to work with the white blood cells and antigens in the blood that go directly to the tumor and attack it.

One of the centers early patients had mesothelioma (cancer in the lining of the lungs), and he was in a lot of pain. After receiving his physical, lab tests, x-rays, biopsy report, and diagnostic, he met with Dr. Rubio. In his consultation, he recommended radiation immediately to help diminish the pain.

The patient said, "Doctor, you are forgetting something. Next week is my birthday. I don't want to do radiation yet, it will deplete my body." Even though Dr. Rubio uses low doses of radiation so that the patient isn't depleted, he respected the patient's wishes and waited two weeks till after his vacation was over. When the patient came back to the hospital and began all the components of treatment, we were able to successfully stop the tumor with radiation combined with the vaccine and oxygen therapies.

If at first our medical team had pushed him into the radiation therapy and not listened to the patient's wants and wishes, he may not have responded as positively. The radiation worked much better when the patient was ready and consented to it. Therein, his body had a positive healing response. (See more patient power stories in chapter 12.)

We hope to express the importance here that patients accept and embrace radiation as a beneficial therapy. Used properly, it can assist to heal cancer quickly and provide support for the body to get well. If you don't want to do radiation as a therapy, then don't accept it. After years of observation, it seems clear, if you do not want a certain therapy and you take it anyway, your brain will block your immune system from receiving positive benefits.

In breaking the cancer code, we have used radiation protocols with one-tenth to one quarter the amounts of standard therapy, sometimes even less, and the response to the radiation combined with the vaccines has been successful. Each patient needs to be assessed individually as to how much radiation and chemotherapy they can handle, and we adjust our low doses accordingly.

Chemotherapy

Early History of Chemotherapy

Chemotherapy was a term coined by German scientist Paul Erhlich, who developed animal models to test the efficacy of various substances (chemicals and antibiotics) in treating various diseases. Chemotherapy was first used in the United States in the early 1900s by researcher George Clowes. Clowes tested various chemicals on cancers that had been transplanted into animals.

From 1906 to 1940, several studies were published describing success in treating tumors in mice with various chemicals. The first chemotherapy used on humans resulted from a wartime accident, in which sailors were accidentally exposed to secret chemical warfare agents during World War II. The seamen were exposed to mustard gas following an explosion. Doctors were amazed to discover their bone marrow and lymph systems depleted following the accidental exposure.

Experimental nitrogen-mustard compounds, called alkylating agents, were used experimentally on cancer patients starting in 1943. Other work on chemotherapies took place at Yale University under wartime secrecy. The original mustard-nitrogen compound proved useful since it killed rapidly growing cells, especially lymphoma cells, but the compound was also extremely toxic and caused severe vomiting and nausea.

By 1950, over five thousand substances had been tested for their usefulness in treating cancer through studies on animals. Many other chemotherapeutic agents have since been developed with positive results as a primary or adjunct treatment to surgery and radiation in traditional medicine.

It is important to remember that all the tests and research done on laboratory animals—rats, guinea pigs, and rabbits—may not necessarily be extrapolated to humans since the animals' cells are so different. Even within the human species, we all have different genes and different DNA codes. We repeatedly reinforce that this is why we need to work on an individual basis with each patient.

Chemotherapy utilizes chemicals to destroy the DNA in cancer cells. The chemotherapy works on rapid-growing cells, which includes most cancers. One of the problems associated with chemotherapy is that it usually is used with no specificity; instead of selectively destroying cancer cells, it attacks all cells in the body that are rapidly growing. Organs with a high rate of cell reproduction and growth are adversely affected. This includes the skin, hair, intestines, and bone marrows. Because of this, cancer patients undergoing chemotherapy typically experience hair loss, skin changes, and diarrhea.

At the same time, we don't need to overuse chemotherapy to the point that patients become adapted and are no longer able to respond to the treatment. Chemotherapy can be used effectively for six or eight months, after which the cancer cells may adapt to it. Our medical team uses specific carriers that combine with the chemotherapy to directly attack the cancer cells and are called IPT (insulin-potentiated therapy). This way we target the chemotherapy to the cancer cells without wasting it on noncancerous cells and can then use a lower dose. In our research, this entire method is effective.

Alternatives to Chemotherapy

Platinum is a natural metal and is very effective to kill rapidly growing cells. We can use the original salt to kill cancer cells, and this can also be used as a very effective carboplatin chemotherapy. We have tested low doses of cisplatin as chemotherapy in conjunction with interferon, interleukin-12, and the active vaccines. Combining these therapies, we have witnessed dramatic changes in tumors and accompanying reductions in tumor sizes. With patients in need, this takes pressure off nerves and diminishes and takes the pain level down.

We also recommend chemo-sensitivity tests to be performed with a patient's tissue to see which responds to the therapy. If a chemo doesn't prove effective, we don't use it. This saves patients the trial of enduring chemos that aren't responsive. Chemotherapies have improved and are getting more specific compared to the past when they were used in a less targeted, generalized form. The most common ways to receive chemotherapy is either orally or through intramuscular or intravenous injections and IVs.

The Downside of Chemotherapy

Not all cancers respond to chemotherapy. According to doctors who have worked with it over the last twenty years, some cancers even grow stronger and become more aggressive when exposed to it. New chemotherapy used in the 1990s became more aggressive.

In many situations, medical doctors will blast cancer with chemotherapies that act within the body like a big atomic bomb. This devastates the patient's whole system and is likely going to poison them. Many use chemotherapy in high doses because it's the primary weapon in their arsenal, and this can negatively affect the whole body.

Many cancers grow in organs that secrete hormones and fluids. When we load chemotherapy into these organs, we're going to weaken the immune system and encourage the tumor cells to become more aggressive. We cannot destroy all the tumor cells with chemotherapy. Cancer cells wait out the effects of chemotherapy by hiding in the glands. Here they will stay hidden until the positive effects of the chemotherapy begin to diminish.

We recommend that instead of using a huge blast of chemo as a single-bullet approach to attacking the cancer itself, a comprehensive approach with chemo as a piece of the puzzle would be better. Some treatment regimens can be so aggressive they don't allow a chance for the patient's body to respond to the chemotherapy before bombarding it with more. The best method we've found is to work with smaller to larger bullets step-by-step in introducing chemotherapy protocols. Our goal is to freeze and stop the tumor from growing and to give the patient health-building protocols, creating an opportunity for the immune system to work.

IPT (insulin-potentiated therapy) and the circadian rhythm are other variables that ensure success. We recommend patients receive chemotherapy when the cancer cells are active. In the pH cycle of the body, the cancer is active from 10:00 a.m. to about 3:00 p.m., when the pH of the body system is acidic. The cancer is more vulnerable to therapies during this time. From 3:00 p.m. to 10:00 p.m., the cancer is usually inactive, and the pH of the system is alkaline. When we applied chemotherapy at a time when the cancer was actively growing and reproducing and metabolizing substances, we have experienced excellent results.

Big controversies have been brewing over twenty years about the use of chemotherapy and radiation. Disappointingly, some chemotherapy initially can cause cancer tumors to shrink, but later the tumors grow back. Many researchers have discovered new chemicals to use for chemotherapy. At the beginning of their studies, they get great benefits (i.e., the chemotherapy reduces the tumor and stops metastasis), but three months later, the cancer starts to grow again.

Why does this happen? From experience, we know that cancer is not static; it's moving and changing all the time and adapting to its environment. The body itself is in constant motion. With our research, we have found that it's best to pretest the cells before using chemotherapy and radiation in specific cancers with specific patients so we know they're going to respond.

There are many chemotherapies that have been used effectively over the years on lymphomas and testicular, oat cell, and squamous cell cancers. In these cases, we need to employ a chemotherapy protocol to help shrink the tumors and give a chance for the immune system to battle fewer cancer cells in the body. But for many other types of cancers, chemotherapy on its own has been ineffective.

Once a tumor is destroyed, the body produces an abundance of uric acid and loses glutamine. Drinking a glass of water with baking soda changes the pH of the body to alkaline and helps the body to eliminate the dead proteins. Ringer's lactate taken in an intravenous infusion helps flush the proteins out of the bloodstream.

By combining chemotherapy, radiation, immunotherapy, and a health-building metabolic program, we see the effects supporting the patient 100 percent. If you are receiving chemotherapy and radiation on a daily basis and are experiencing negative side effects, you should know that there are other effective alternatives. Research shows that radiation stays in the body for a month and needs to not be repeated every day.

Breaking the cancer code works as a multifaceted approach. We have been blessed to see remarkable healings and the shrinking of a variety of tumors with a very good quality of life reestablished for so many patients after these treatments.

Sometimes, doctors who are using chemotherapy and radiation will tell patients to stop all vitamins and minerals! You must realize how vitamins and minerals support the body; they are a nutritional insurance to protect and support your immune system. We hope that thorough education, we will inspire patients to get more assertive at health building and detoxification while going through their cancer treatment. We see this as a pivotal point of breaking the cancer code.

Helping Patients Embrace, Not Fear, Treatment

We want to educate patients to eliminate the fear of radiation and chemotherapy because these therapies can be most effective. When your medical staff come from the perspective of respect for patients and work together as a team, these methods can help, not harm, the patient. You should not be afraid of these two words: *chemotherapy* and *radiation*. These two treatments can support you in your healing process, if you believe they will. If you react with fear to any therapy, the body can potentially suffer more from this resistance.

In conjunction with all the vaccines, we incorporate a strong detoxification program to expedite the removal of the dead cancer cells and protein by-products from the body. We also use the Rife frequency generator to maintain control over the tumor. We will offer more on our extensive detoxification protocols in the next chapter, which we see help people get their vitality back during and after cancer.

Chapter 5

The Importance of Cancer Detoxification

With all the variables to successful cancer healing, none is more important than cleaning up the battlefield (i.e., patient's body) as the cancer war wages on. When a cancer patient receives anticancer therapies—such as chemotherapy, radiation, herbs, supplements, and more—millions of cancer cells are destroyed. Along with these dead cells, millions of dead proteins float throughout the body. These dead proteins overload the extracellular fluids in the blood and place adverse pressure on the remaining healthy cells. Unless this condition is dealt with quickly, normal cells will starve because they cannot sustain normal metabolic and chemical reactions in such a polluted environment.

When dead proteins produce more free radicals, the result is cell autointoxication. Oftentimes, patients will be told that they have no evidence of the disease, but they still don't feel quite right. This is because the cells need to be flushed and detoxified of these harmful toxins. Without supportive measures, the body attempts to remove the toxins through normal elimination channels. If these channels are overloaded, an excessively toxic patient may experience hair loss, nail loss, vomiting, diarrhea, and blood disorders just from the toxins alone!

Detoxification techniques are essential tools that allow the body to effectively eliminate dead tumor cells and proteins, as well as the toxic effects of some cancer therapies. Simultaneously as we detoxify the patient, we give the body's natural defenses a better opportunity to work effectively. We try not to overload the immune system by attempting to perform too many functions simultaneously. Instead, we encourage people to incorporate detoxification practices while dealing with both live and dead cancer cells.

As part of breaking the cancer code, we need to stop the tumors and stop the pain. When patients don't respond, we know to work harder and more intelligently. Detoxification techniques offer valuable tools to strengthen our natural immunity in our quest to control cancer.

Detoxification helps prevent healthy cells from becoming overloaded with toxins so they can continue to function and sustain normal metabolic reactions. When a cell reacts metabolically, it uses nutrients to complete a specific function. After the reaction, the cell produces toxins or residuals. If we don't remove these residuals, the cell and surrounding tissues will be damaged. When cells are bathed with toxins from the outside, such as from chemicals in body-care products or preservatives in foods, and then add to that radiation, the cells can become overloaded and subsequently die.

The simple technique we use counteracts autointoxication and supports the body marvelously to keep patients functioning and stable. Throughout this book, we emphasize suggestions like this one so you can benefit from integrating detoxification protocols and cancer treatments no matter what cancer therapy you choose.

Throughout the body, organs work in balance and need to be supported to assist them in detoxifying the body. These organs include the lungs, colon, liver, skin, kidneys, and lymphatic system, which all function to eliminate metabolic wastes. These organs cleanse us internally and work together to maintain a harmonious balance in the body as they eliminate dead cancer, dead proteins, and chemicals from the body. Let's take a look at each one and how we can effectively cleanse them.

The Lungs

The lungs help balance pH (acid/alkaline) levels in the blood. They play an important role in cancer treatment because they release built-up toxicity in the system. They also work with the blood to oxygenate and transport oxygen to the cells. The blood delivers oxygen through its hemoglobin. Oxygen molecules bind temporarily with ionized iron molecules in the hemoglobin, which then releases oxygen at the cellular level. The carbon monoxide produced through the process of cell metabolism is carried back to the lungs primarily as blood-soluble bicarbonate ions and then released as carbon dioxide when we exhale.

We can accelerate the toxin-removing function of the lungs by using different medications to push oxygen to the cells and recharge them. Introducing beneficial medications—such as zinc, germanium, and low doses of interferon—into the oxygen given to patients will help their immune system attack the cancer. We gain the benefits of using interferon in this treatment modality with none of the negative side effects.

Another method that increases oxygenation is "deep breathing" where we have patients breathe oxygen twenty times in fifteen seconds. Normal respiration occurs fourteen to sixteen times per minute. This technique quickly removes about 1 percent of the blood's general toxicity and helps it to release toxins faster, including those found in chemicals from chemotherapy, radiation, or dead proteins from dead cells. With this method, toxins are immediately flushed out of the blood.

In breaking the cancer code, we prescribe the use of deep-breathing three times a day for ten minutes and an additional ten minutes just before patients go to sleep. This treatment helps the lungs to quickly remove toxicity and better oxygenate the blood. The treatment dramatically increases the chances of breaking cancer's anaerobic growth cycle.

The Colon

Also known as the large intestine, the colon is a coiled tube, about five feet long, with extensive surface areas that efficiently digest foods and absorb beneficial substances.

The colon has two functions—absorption and excretion.

The colon performs the vital role of absorbing water and salts from food contents passing through it and returning them to the bloodstream. If material passes too quickly through the colon, water is inadequately absorbed, and the result is diarrhea. Unchecked, diarrhea can dangerously dehydrate the body, and the subsequent loss of salts can be fatal.

The opposite problem—an unusually slow journey of materials through the colon and excessive water reabsorption—can result in a hard mass of undigested materials and constipation. Cleansing techniques such as colonics, colemas, and enemas have been used for many years to assist the excretion and elimination processes, as well as to help the body absorb beneficial substances. Substances that contact the walls of the colon are absorbed quickly and rapidly into the bloodstream.

As an organ of detoxification, the colon will work continuously to collect and eliminate dead cancer cells or dead proteins and the chemicals from chemotherapy. We want to keep the colon in constant movement through natural laxatives, so we use fibers from fruits and plants to raise the level of peristalsis.

At Rubio Cancer Center, we use a lot of fiber in the diet to help absorb and wash chemicals out. Chemicals have a tendency to attach to the DNA of the cells of the colon's walls, which we don't want. Fiber helps to pick up chemicals and flush them out, giving the colon a better chance of avoiding the development of cancer.

Many natural health practitioners believe that disease begins in the digestive system and colon. Benefits of cleansing the colon include detoxifying the blood, cleansing the bloodstream, and stimulating the internal organs. The colon is highly absorbent with whatever is inside it, which is why we introduce beneficial medications that will assist in detoxifying the blood.

Enemas as Treatment

An enema is a technique through which we can introduce water and medications into the colon. We usually place sixteen to twenty-two ounces of water and beneficial medications (i.e., colostrum, shark cartilage, maitake mushroom, or coffee) into an enema bucket. A line runs from the bucket to a plastic tube that we gently insert into the rectum and large intestine. Enemas can help the body absorb all the medications and at the same time stimulate the colon to eliminate residue and wastes. They also help absorb residual radiation and facilitate the quick release of any dead cancer cells from the colon, liver, and lymphatic system.

These suggested enemas are absorbed 60 percent through the intestinal wall and introduced into the bloodstream. These preparations then travel directly to the liver and on to the entire metabolic system. If patients have ascites or fluid in the colon, lungs, or heart, they can still use enemas with caution. Since the amount of water is very small, they won't absorb too much but will still get all the benefits of these medications.

Specific Enemas

We offer different types of enemas for different types of cancer. For specific cancers of the digestive tract, we recommend colostrums, which contain gamma globulin. Gamma globulin enhances immune system functioning and stops inflammation caused by cancer in the colon, digestive tract, liver, stomach, esophagus, and tongue. When these enemas are given every day, cancer tumors start shrinking.

We recommend mushroom enemas for patients who have lymphomas, leukemia, and brain tumors. Shiitake mushrooms, called the King of the Mushrooms, are used for these enemas. This is also a popular supplement, and we can also eat them as part of an anticancer diet. Maitake mushrooms effectively diminish and stop tumor activities. They create a fungal environment within the body that competes with cancer cells for nutrition and helps to starve tumors.

For all types of tumors, we suggest enemas that contain shark cartilage. Patients can administer shark cartilage enemas on a daily basis, and the result we see is tumors stop growing, and it can stop the metastasis of cancer. The cartilage contains a substance called mucopolysaccharide that stops angiogenesis and doesn't allow the tumor to stimulate the surrounding tissue to make new blood vessels, which nourish it. The tumor stabilizes because it becomes encapsulated and quits growing.

A favorite for years are coffee enemas as they are the best way to flush toxins from the liver, lungs, and brain. The caffeine in coffee produces a general stimulant to the system and makes the organs work faster. Since the colon is directly connected to the liver, it is an excellent way to transport substances to the liver.

Medications in enemas are especially beneficial when patients are unable to take supplements by mouth. In this case, we want to apply megadoses of medications to the body. The prescriptive enemas are also useful when patients have fluid retention since they can more quickly respond to the supplements and medications provided through an enema.

We don't employ colonic therapy when patients have water in their stomachs or lungs since it puts more pressure on their systems, making it more difficult to get back into balance. Enemas are a safer alternative for these patients than colonics since they use smaller amounts of water. The patient will still get the full benefit of the supplements or medications added.

Use Enemas Only under a Doctor's Supervision

Enemas should be used only under a doctor's supervision or through someone specifically trained to administer them. In orthodox medicine, enemas are used in hospitals as laxatives for constipated patients, and they must be given under the supervision of an MD or a naturopathic doctor. Before using enemas, the patient should consult a doctor for information on correct applications and possible side effects.

Excessive use of enemas can cause the colon to become lazy or dependent on them for facilitating bowel movements. We avoid this problem, which is known as lazy bowel syndrome. We normally administer enemas every other day for the first month, three times a week for the second month, two times a week for the third month, and once a week from the fourth month onward. The colon should start working normally after that. It should be noted that, after decades of helping patients heal, we have seen no negative side effects from the use of these enemas.

Our Enema Program

As a part of our cancer therapy, once patients are released from the hospital, they are instructed to use retention enemas three days a week with a break on Sundays.

On Mondays, Wednesdays, and Fridays, we recommend a coffee retention enema, which consists of sixteen ounces of very warm water, two teaspoons of prepared coffee, and twenty drops of hydrogen peroxide.

For patients with colon and digestive tumors, we suggest the use of colostrum enemas, with sixteen ounces of very warm water mixed with two teaspoons of colostrum. For patients with colon, prostate, or lung cancer; lymphoma; or leukemia, we use mushroom enemas, with sixteen ounces of very warm water mixed with the mushrooms.

Once a week, a shark retention enema is given for all types of tumors. When we give an enema in the clinic, we may include a tablespoon of shark, bovine, or snake cartilage with sixteen ounces of water. The cartilage contains mucopolysaccharide, which stops the growth of cancer and is absorbed through the walls of the colon. For the home program, the formula is eight ounces of very warm water mixed with two teaspoons of shark powder.

Procedures:

There are many positions for patients to take when giving themselves an enema. One of the best is laying on the side with knees bent toward the chest and a towel underneath to catch any spillage. A two-quart bag should be used and can be hung from a towel rack, or a hot-water bottle can be laid on a sink counter. The bag should be higher than one foot above the buttocks. Water should be five degrees warmer than body temperature and should be taken until it needs to be eliminated.

Colonics

Colonics require a special machine that regulates the amount of water released into and out of the colon. The patient relaxes comfortably on his/her back on a padded board and is told to breathe deeply. A line runs from the machine, and a sterilized speculum is coated with petroleum jelly, calendula gel or K-Y Jelly can be used as a sterile lubricant. The therapist tells the patient to create pressure like a bowel movement as the tube is gently inserted into the anus. The patient feels no discomfort with this method.

The colon is then gently flushed with warm water and beneficial supplements. With colonics, the patient's colon is cleaned out, and medications are absorbed at the same time. We have used herbs, ozone, supplements, cartilage, coffee, red clover, or pau d'arco teas; all have been part of our protocol, administered into the colon along with the water. Ozone added to the colonic introduces more oxygen to the cells and helps to break the anaerobic cycle of cancer.

The colon therapist will often gently massage the colon during the filling and releasing processes by rubbing the abdomen. As the water is expelled, a glass tube may allow the viewing and collection of the materials released.

Colonics can be used as a part of detoxification therapy, but not all cancer patients are advised to undergo it. It is contraindicated for patients that have fluids in their abdomen, lungs or an obstruction or bypass. Using colonics in these instances will add too much pressure and water to the patient's system. Instead, these patients should use an enema to receive the benefits of colon detoxification. A colonic should be employed only once or twice a week so the patient does not become dependent on the colonic for elimination.

Colonics support the other organs of detoxification by helping to remove dead metabolic proteins and the normal and dead flora from the intestines.

Colonics allow us to create a new environment in the colon, and once completed, probiotics are added to recover the normal flora and to replace the friendly bacteria that may have been lost.

We also want to mention something important that health practitioners want to address: it's to administer *acidophilus*, vitamin C, and minerals as an implant after a colonic to recreate healthy balanced environments of flora in their patients' colons.

At a minimum, the colon should produce a bowel movement once or twice a day. A colonic will empty the colon of wastes that include dead proteins from dead cancer cells and those generated by normal metabolism. In some patients, harmful bacteria grow on the dead proteins in the colon. Colonics help patients to stop this bacterial growth by flushing it out.

Colonics are also used to absorb beneficial substances—60 to 75 percent of all water, supplements, and medications are absorbed into the bloodstream through the use of colonics. The colon absorbs water but also releases it over the course of the colonic. During colonics, water and supplements are absorbed into the bloodstream. The normal process of osmosis prevents the extra water in the bloodstream from entering cells throughout the body. Afterward, the colon works with the liver, lungs, kidneys, skin, and lymph system to release excess water from the system.

About five gallons of water are used over the course of a colonic. We've seen patients eliminate big ropes of mucus, toxicity, dead tumor cells, and sometimes parasites. Once the big ropes are eliminated, the process of healing accelerates. Colonics are an important tool in dealing with cancer because this therapy supports all the others by removing the pressure of dead cancer cells from the body. Colonics are a popular therapy among natural healers, but it is important to emphasize once again that patients use the services of experienced professionals when receiving a colonic.

Colemas

A colema consists of five gallons of water in a bucket to which a tube or line is attached. At the end of the line is a catheter that is inserted into the rectum. Water flows into the rectum with the normal pressure of gravity and passes through a special bulb that checks inflow and outflow. Shark cartilage and herbs—such as pau d'arco, chaparral, or cat's claw—can be added to the water.

A colema is good therapy to treat any type of cancer patient except those who have fluid in the abdomen (ascites), fluid in the lungs, edema (swelling), or some obstruction in the colon. Colemas clean dead proteins and waste materials from the colon and, at the same time, help the body to absorb the added beneficial herbs and medications. Colemas can be used three times a week for a month. After a colema, the patient's colon needs to return to normal, so the friendly bacteria, enzymes, minerals, and vitamin C that may have been lost are replaced through an implant.

Lymphatic System

The lymphatic system is an integral part of our immune system—our natural defense mechanism. In addition to filtering foreign substances and cell wastes from the blood, it also stores white blood cells called lymphocytes. When white blood cells devour dead proteins and chemicals in the bloodstream, the lymph nodes ingest the foreign bodies and work with the liver and kidneys to eliminate them from the system.

The lymphatic system functions through a series of capillaries, vessels, and ducts that absorb excess fluids from the tissues. The capillaries are closed on one end and join together with other capillaries on the other end to form vessels that empty into ducts. The lymphatic system is passive and relies on a network of valves and pressure created by the body's movements to propel it along.

Once the extracellular fluids are absorbed, they are cleansed of bacteria, proteins, and chemicals. The filtered and cleansed fluids are then returned to the bloodstream. For all of us, and especially cancer patients, it is important to keep the lymphatic system open, moving, and circulating the lymph. In some cases, a special lymphatic drainage massage is given to help the system function at a higher level.

The most important part of the lymphatic system is located in the chest, the thoracic duct. Simply by breathing harder, we allow the lymph to move. Also by moving our body—just by walking and breathing—we help it to eliminate dead cancer cells. Contraction of the skeletal muscles helps the lymph to move along. While a patient is passively sitting in a chair or lying in a hospital bed, the lymph is not moving fast enough to be able to quickly eliminate the dead cancer cells and dead proteins.

In a patient who has cancer, the lymphatic system removes dead cancer cells, and they pass through the bloodstream to the kidneys, colon, and skin, where they are eliminated from the system through the urine, excrement, and sweat. To stimulate lymphatic functioning, we employ specific formulas derived from beans called fito enatogrutinina. Other therapies, such as specific amino acids combined with mineral supplements and electrolytes, also help to stimulate lymphatic circulation.

Lymphomas, tumors that grow in the lymphatic system, make it difficult for the lymph system to drain. When cancer tumors start shrinking in these areas, the lymphatic system needs special support to begin to properly function again.

Infections cause the lymph nodes to swell and become inflamed because the immune system can't control the excess dead proteins. If patients notice that their lymph glands are enlarged for more than fourteen days, they should see a doctor who will look for signs of viruses, AIDS, herpes, or bacterial infections or cancer. As part of cancer therapy, we want to keep the lymphatic system functioning continuously to support the body to eliminate dead cancer cells.

The Liver

The liver, the body's largest gland and second-largest organ, performs a myriad of vital functions. It produces liver juices, and the gallbladder produces bile to break up chemicals and antigens that may appear in the digestive tract. The liver has a vital metabolic role, metabolizing the carbohydrates, fats, and proteins from foods. The liver also acts as a filter by eliminating foreign substances from the blood. Other roles of the liver include destroying worn-out blood cells and producing the factors that assist the blood to clot.

The liver is composed of highly vascular tissue, meaning it contains many blood vessels. The liver receives most of its blood supply from the portal vein, which transports digested nutrients and hormones from the intestines, hormones from the pancreas, and substances from the spleen. The liver receives the other 25 percent of its blood supply from the hepatic artery. Hepatic veins return blood from the liver to the heart. Because of this unique circulatory route, 100 percent of every medication absorbed by the colon arrives directly at the liver. In the detoxification process, any colonics, colemas, and enemas that cleanse the colon also serve to detoxify or clean the liver as well.

Coffee enemas are an especially effective technique that increases liver function, stimulating it to cleanse itself of deposits, all without negative side effects. The caffeine in coffee stimulates the liver to produce more liver juices and bile. The body, in turn, starts making more hormones, which will affect cancer growth. To counteract this system-stimulating activity, hormone blockers can be employed to stop the cancer growth.

For patients suffering from hepatitis, the inflammation is diminished through coffee enemas. After the caffeine causes the liver cells to empty themselves, they start functioning normally again.

When treating liver cancer, we can inject substances directly into its artery for maximum effectiveness. We recommend specific medications such as carbamide combined with low doses of chemotherapy. We can also use alcohol injected into the tumor area, which causes the tumor to diminish. In Dr. Rubio's work utilizing these therapies, liver tumors have been dramatically reduced, and the memory restored for normal healthy liver cells, not cancer cells, has been revived to grow and flourish.

Regenerating the Liver

Even with a minimum of 1 to 5 percent of functioning liver cells, the liver can regenerate to 40 to 50 percent of its former capacity. A well-functioning liver is essential to a balanced metabolism. Fortunately, the liver is able to regenerate itself after being injured or diseased. If a disease progresses beyond the tissue's capacity to regenerate new cells, the body's entire metabolism is severely affected. To regenerate a damaged liver, we have several treatments and techniques. We may have the patient drink two ounces of raw liver juice combined with two ounces of grape juice. We also may apply human growth hormone or synthetic growth hormones from salmon to the liver on a daily basis. This allows the liver to be nourished with all the amino acids necessary for its cells to reproduce, regenerating the entire organ.

Other substances taken orally are also beneficial for liver regeneration. These include chromium, which stops inflammation, and milk thistle extract, which helps with the rejuvenation process.

While the liver is regenerating, it is important to let it rest so no proteins or fats are allowed in the diet for ten days. This allows the liver to take a break from some of its digestive functions so it can heal itself. A healthy liver, vital to a balanced metabolism, will support the immune system so it can deal with cancer more effectively.

The Skin

The skin is the body's largest organ. It protects the internal organs and systems while it senses and interacts with the outside environment. The skin protects our bodies from infection by bacteria, viruses, parasites, and fungi. The skin regulates body temperature through a system of complex interactions between the layers of fat and sweat glands and the constriction of blood vessels. When challenged by threatening substances or environments, the skin can produce several allergic reactions, including redness, swelling, and pain—all signs of inflammation.

Two functions of the skin are absorption and excretion. The skin absorbs water and all other substances put on it, including creams, petroleum products, cosmetics, perfumes, bath products, and chemicals from contact with bedding and clothes. When we perspire, the body excretes the broken-down proteins of dead cancer cells and the chemicals from chemotherapy. It is important to support the elimination processes of the skin to keep it highly functioning.

The skin is the largest organ that eliminates toxins, and the quicker and better it does its job, the faster the healing process. For patients undergoing chemotherapy or radiation, we've developed techniques to assist the skin in eliminating the accompanying toxins caused by the therapies. A specific enzyme, alpha glykerol, is contained in green cabbage. The patient can drink green cabbage juice to remove the toxins from chemotherapy and radiation and assist the skin in helping with this process.

For the cancer patient, it is especially important to keep the skin clean. Using filtered drinking water and bathwater is essential to avoid possible negative effects from chlorine, fluoride, and free radicals in ordinary tap water. Skin brushes can be used to stimulate circulation and further release dead skin cells. We also recommend hot baths containing baking soda, sea salts, and ginger to encourage the release of toxins through the skin, along with herbs such as chamomile. These simple techniques keep the skin in good condition with its pH and oils in balance.

We know that chemicals are absorbed into the bloodstream through the skin, so we take note and break the cancer code, using organic and biodegradable soap. We know that dyes and chemicals are also toxic, so we suggest white blankets and bed linens because we don't want chemicals from dyes to contact the skin. The same rule applies to toilet paper. We advise our patients to avoid aluminum-containing deodorants, hair coloring, and chemical perfumes. There are many natural-source cosmetics and perfumes made from aloe vera plants, essential oils, and flower sources.

Taking these precautions, we prevent patients' bodies from becoming more intoxicated through their skin. We similarly protect them from toxins in the air they breathe through the use of air filters. While in the healing process, it's important to not overload the immune system with millions of unnecessary synthetic chemicals in the bloodstream.

As part of our therapy, patients are instructed to take daily hot baths to aid the detoxification process through the skin. As mentioned earlier, we use a detoxification ginger bath recipe, see page 152 for further instructions, which includes three-fourth cup of Dead Sea or pink sea salts combined with ginger and baking soda. We also recommend that patients only wash with organic vegetable soaps or glycerin bars, being sure the soaps don't have petroleum products or parabens. The natural soaps we suggest does not cause bathtub rings, burning eyes nor changes to the natural pH of the skin.

Taking too many baths a day will weaken patients. Staying in the tub too long will also cause weakness. Soaking for fourteen minutes in a very hot tub of water once each day is sufficient. We make sure a patient wets their face, neck, and chest. Turning over in the tub is advised if possible. If a patient feels light-headed or dizzy, placing cold washcloths on the head and the back of the neck should take care of the problem. Patients are advised to be careful not to get a chill after their bath, to dry off completely, and to cover themselves afterward.

Kidneys

Through the urinary tract, the kidneys excrete excess water, potassium, sodium and chloride, and urea and uric acid—the toxic wastes of metabolic processes. Millions of units in the kidneys, called nephrons, filter the blood and collect and eliminate wastes. The kidneys also eliminate toxins from drugs and their breakdown products. The kidneys stimulate the body to produce red blood cells, increase absorption of oxygen, and control blood pressure. The kidneys maintain the water balance and acidity of the blood.

Along with the lungs, the kidneys are the organs that keep the body's pH in the metabolism in balance along with regulating the levels of good proteins in the bloodstream. In cancer patients, the pH level in the blood becomes acidic, causing the internal organs to become partially disabled. A by-product of cancer cell metabolism is lactic acid since cancer cells don't utilize oxygen. It is this lactic acid that breaks the membranes of the kidneys and causes the pH to become unbalanced. In our cancer therapies, we flush the kidneys to switch the bloodstream's pH. This helps the other organs to maintain an ideal environment for healthy cell metabolism.

Our simple therapy is for patients to drink eight glasses of water daily that contain bicarbonate or baking soda to flush the kidneys. This technique will switch the pH in the blood and immune system and get the body moving and working again.

When the pH is acidic in the bloodstream, the body's cells get a jellylike environment surrounding them, and the white blood cells are unable to move through the extracellular fluids. Natural supplements to ingest to assist kidney function include barley greens, alfalfa, spirulina algae, lemon seeds, and oranges. Drinking good corn silk teas also helps. All these items flush the kidneys and keep its filters functioning on a higher level. We drink a lot of water to flush out toxins and not allow the blood to get thicker since it is already overloaded with dead proteins and broken membranes floating through it. We want to prevent the patient from becoming weaker.

When the lactic acid produced by cancer cells causes cell membranes to break in the kidneys, proteins escape into the extracellular fluids, and the patient gets weaker. Edema (swelling) can result at the same time. While undergoing cancer therapies, patients need the support of the kidneys to maintain an alkaline environment and assist the immune system in fighting cancer.

Breast Cancer Detoxification Scenario

As an example of how all these organs work together to eliminate toxicity, suppose a patient has breast cancer. Traditional medical doctors would perform a mastectomy, lymphadenectomy, and adenectomy. Then radiation therapy would be used, along with chemotherapy and hormone therapy.

The patient has just lost (1) one gland (the breast) and (2) part of the lymphatic system, including ten to twenty lymph nodes, and (3) has received toxic doses of radiation and chemotherapy. The radiation and chemotherapy destroys a lot of cells, not just cancer.

These dead cells are now floating through the body, waiting for it to eliminate them. If the organs of elimination are abnormally functioning, the dead proteins and chemicals will overtax the immune system, and the patient will experience the side effects of autointoxication, which may include vomiting, diarrhea, and skin burns. If patients use detoxification therapies before chemotherapy or radiation, our experience is they won't vomit or experience as many problems with their skins. This is because the organs of elimination will be cleansed beforehand and are likely to be working effectively to release the toxicity once treatment begins. Most of our patients undergo several days of detoxification before we get started on their therapies.

Protection against Autointoxication

Here is an example of how we utilize green cabbage as part of our detoxification protocol and a description of how this simple therapy works for patients undergoing radiation or chemotherapy:

1) The patient drinks a glass of green cabbage juice before receiving radiation. Green cabbage contains an enzyme that protects some of the noncancerous cells from becoming toxic and also protects the kidneys and liver.
2) A green cabbage poultice is applied to the site of the radiation so the skin will not be as likely to burn.
3) A specific bath containing baking soda, ginger, and sea salts will protect the skin and remove toxicity caused by the radiation.
4) While receiving radiation and chemotherapy, the patient will breathe a special geranium formula to exchange toxins for oxygen and quickly remove the dead cells.
5) Specific formulas and IVs specially customized to the patient will protect cells and remove toxicity.

Peristalsis needs to be maintained in the colon to flush out dead cancer cells by employing enemas, colonics, and colemas. We need to keep the kidneys and liver working twenty-four hours a day to eliminate cancer cells. Thus, if a patient receives the traditional oncological treatments of radiation and chemotherapy, he will get the benefits of the therapies without the negative side effects.

During treatment, we advise a minimum of one enema, colonic, or colema per week. Water can be mixed with chaparral, red clover tea, pau d'arco, cat's claw, or cuachalalate. Because plain water can irritate the bowels, one to two ounces of flaxseed tea or bentonite clay can be mixed into a gallon of water. The best water to use is reverse osmosis water or, at least, filtered water to remove the chlorine and other chemicals that may be present. The water temperature should be about five degrees warmer than body temperature. Here is an easy way to make flaxseed tea: soak seeds overnight in warm water, then strain off the seeds in the morning, and you've got flaxseed tea.

Detoxification is one of the first steps taken to remove cancer from the body. We tell our patients that the detoxification process alone is not strong enough to remove the tumor but serves to excellently support the other cancer therapies we provide.

Using a detoxification regimen, we make it easier for the immune system to eliminate dead cancer cells and chemicals. The patient's immune system will only be burdened with eliminating hundreds of cells a day instead of the millions eliminated by those undergoing traditional treatments. We've seen good results when this method is used in conjunction with metabolic therapy and immunotherapy, as well as the traditional methods of chemotherapy and radiation.

In patients with cancers of the colon, skin, lungs, brain, liver, and breast—as well as lymphoma, sarcoma, and leukemia—we've seen the tumors' growths stopped or their sizes reduced. And when we combine all these therapies, the tumors oftentimes disappear completely.

Chelation

We use chelation to remove toxins caused by chemotherapy and radiation from the bloodstream using EDTA. When applied through an IV directly to the veins, the chelation formula of vitamins, minerals, and chemicals (called EDTA) facilitates the removal of dead cancer cells, proteins, chemicals, radiation, and metals from the bloodstream. These are filtered through the kidneys and eliminated through the urine.

Following chelation, we need to replace the beneficial substances lost through an IV infusion of minerals, vitamins, and other health-sustaining nutrients.

Medicinal Teas

Cuachalalate and pau d'arco teas both work to detoxify the bloodstream. They help to restore the internal organs to normal functioning through affecting the alkaline/phosphates levels. They help protect the healthy organs and stop cancer growth. They have been used not only for curing cancer but for other diseases as well.

Pau d'arco seems to protect the liver even when the patient is undergoing chemotherapy, with the theory that the healthy cells will outlast the cancer cells. Pau d'arco helps to prevent nausea, keeps the hair from falling out, protects the eyesight so the eyes don't fail, keeps the bowels moving so they keep doing their job, and keeps functioning the immune system. Consequently, another benefit of these teas and detoxification protocols is patients get less pneumonia, tuberculosis, or other killer diseases when their immune systems fail because their body is working so hard to fight off the effects of chemotherapy.

With chemotherapy, the first organ to be compromised is the liver, whose main jobs are to detoxify the bloodstream and to regulate the body's metabolism. The second organs to be adversely affected are the kidneys, which filter out the poisons.

A Simple Detoxification Method

Here's information for a patient and doctor about a simple detoxification method:

1) Drink eight glasses of water per day. Add some sodium bicarbonate, an antacid, to the water early in the day to avoid any blockage in the kidneys.
2) Drink a natural laxative (one tablespoon of cascara sagrada and psyllium plants mixed with apple juice or water) three times per day.

The constant use of detoxification procedures helps patients in the healing process. We also recommend drinking a lot of water with sodium bicarbonate added to avoid any blockage in the kidneys caused by dead proteins.

In breaking the cancer code, we want to stop using narcotics as painkillers as much as possible because they shut down the organs of detoxification, including the liver, kidneys, colon, and lungs. It's difficult for the body to heal when its internal systems are shut down. We'll discuss the use of different types of painkillers in chapter 9, "Nature Power."

Rubio Cancer Center Home Program

When our patients are released from the hospital, they go home and continue their healing with the home program. At the end of chapter 12, we provide a specific outline of the home program. See "Prevention Power." However, we want to review a few of the recommendations here.

Chapter 6

How to Use Your Diet to Heal

Once a person has been diagnosed with cancer, the idea of eating healthy is no longer an option. In order for their body (a.k.a. life vehicle) to function and heal, the fuel now has to be premium, and the maintenance of the vehicle is daily. Never has diet been more important than when healing a condition like cancer.

The foods and drinks we ingest give us energy and the tools we need for our cells to function efficiently and harmoniously. In today's standard American diet (SAD) with heavily processed foods, the very substances designed to nourish us can cause our organs to malfunction and make us sick. For many years, food was ignored as a cancer-causing agent.

Doctors know today that certain foods can be initiators for cancer and other illnesses. Our bodies are harmed by foods containing preservatives, antibiotics, and pesticides, to name a few. The many forms of sugar—from modified high-fructose corn syrup to pure cane syrup to brown rice syrup to agave nectar—all make foods tastier as they stimulate appetite and cancer cells. Because the standard American lifestyle is rush-rush-rush with little time to relax, many of us eat and chew our foods improperly, which means we absorb less of the nutrients available in what we consume. Cancer healing is a wake-up call to make changes in many of these areas.

Nature's Pharmacy

Our bodies contain all the enzymes they need to break down the foods we eat and to properly absorb them. But sometimes these enzymes fail to function when they encounter certain foods or chemicals, in the way food is processed, that make the digestive system unable to break them down properly. This results in little to no nutritional support at all.

Many doctors work with specific diets to try to arrest cancer, and it is sometimes very difficult for them to choose the right diet for each individual patient. Some doctors get excellent results, while others have minor, or insignificant results because their patients each possess different genes, plus each individual responds differently to different foods. One person might function best on a diet of raw vegetables and smoothies; another might prefer heavier meals with legumes and grains. There are endless combinations, too numerous to mention here.

Healing Cancer with Diet

Some of the dietary plans used to treat illness and cancer have been vegetarian, macrobiotic, alkaline, and fasting diets. We suggest that the best way to choose a diet is to know the patient's genes and body. This will help the doctor to prescribe a revised and improved approach to a proper diet specific for the patient.

The type of diet chosen is an important factor in fighting cancer because the type of nutrition the body receives can slow down or stop the growth of cancer cells. All metabolic reactions in the cells depend on the presence of certain nutrients and water. By using the technique of matching patients' blood types with diet, we help stop cancer cells from growing and transform them to normal cells.

At many health centers and cancer centers, including ours, we use diets that are determined by blood type and don't put additional stress on the patient's body. Cancer patients are already under tremendous stress, and their diets should create harmony and not add challenges to their bodies. We have seen tremendous benefits and positive results by incorporating more plant-based, nutrient-dense, and whole-food-specialized diets into their treatment plans and lifestyles.

There is a huge movement in the United States toward these healthier preservative—and sugar-free diets that open up a whole new lifestyle. One of the best companies leading the way is Whole Foods Market. Carolyn has directly experienced this company's commitment to keeping their employees healthy with health immersion programs. Both she and her husband, Bryan, were privileged to attend a health immersion program which focused on the importance of nutrient-rich food and lifestyle solutions. Since today there are so many sweeteners added and oils too that make foods addictive, eating fresh and healthy has never been more important.

The standard American diet has been omnivorous (i.e., we consume both animal and vegetable products). We actually do need to eat a wide variety of foods that contain proteins, carbohydrates, and lipids to keep our bodies functioning well. That is the purpose of nutrition! We also know that the fast-food society has taken a toll on most of us. Now, when patients need to heal, a dietary regimen for cancer patients should take into account the genetic constitution of the patient.

Plant-Based, Nutrient-Rich Foods

During treatment and even after treatment is finished, the diet should avoid stressing and upsetting the hemodynamics of the blood and avoid rapid changes in the hemoglobin. The type of diet for cancer patients is important because cells need nutrients, water, and oxygen to function and achieve homeostasis.

Patients with blood type A or B, positive or negative, can be vegetarians, vegans, and the like, without having problems producing hemoglobin or with bouts of anemia. Patients with these blood types usually have enough selenium (an antioxidant) in their systems and do not require additional animal protein in their diets. They can also obtain the negative electrical charges useful in fighting cancer from ingesting vegetables alone.

These patients usually know from experience that they crave their veggies and grains while not so much the traditional proteins. As with all things plant based, A and B blood types have to be cautious with fats and sweets because sometimes eating "so healthy" means finding a treat. They will traditionally find their treats with fats and sweets.

In healing cancer, the hemoglobin is complex, and most people who aren't blood type A or B don't have the time and energy to figure out every little grain, nut, and seed composition for their hemodynamics. So for patients like blood type O, we offer a different solution.

Not All Cancer Patients Can Be Vegetarians

After years of research, we have found that not all cancer patients can be vegetarians because their bodies do require animal proteins to produce hemoglobin. Patients with O-positive or O-negative blood types require animal protein to form hemoglobin and to facilitate cellular functioning.

The best sources of protein are shark and organically grown chicken raised with no hormones or chemicals. Organically grown turkey is good as well, along with any kind of fish except salmon and tuna. *Organic* is a very important word; it means antibiotic-free. Salmon and tuna are the most popular fish we eat; unfortunately, they are loaded with mercury, one of the causes of prostate, breast, and bladder cancer. Patients with O-type blood also need to consume liver, which provides selenium. Liver, along with other antioxidants, produces a negative electrical charge within the system that enhances metabolic functioning. This is going to slow down the tumor's growth since tumors like to grow in a positively charged environment. It is our experience that patients with an O-positive or negative blood type need to eat a small amount of animal protein as well as a nutrient-rich, plant-based diet.

Starving the Cancer and Feeding the Body

Taking the blood type into account, a cancer diet is specifically formulated to provide nutrition to the body and its functions while denying nutrition to the tumor. Patients with tumoral activities are in a state of cachexia (i.e., their bodies degenerate and lose protein and organ mass while the cancer grows). What is cachexia? It is a process of cellular destruction, which occurs because tumor cells are stealing nutrients from the body.

We know that tumor cells grow in dextrorotation, meaning that the DNA rotates to the right as the cells reproduce. Subsequently, we starve the tumor while nourishing the healthy cells with nutrients and medications that rotate to the left. Some examples are levulose acids switched to the left side, lipids with a negative polarization, and glucose that rotates to the left. All these substances nourish the body, not the tumor.

Cancer patients need more nutrients, proteins, carbohydrates, lipids, minerals, vitamins, and enzymes in their diets than do noncancer patients because cancer cells take and monopolize all the nutrients from their bodies. The cancer cells grow through the process of fermentation. They don't need oxygen to survive, and they milk all the glucose and proteins from the body and produce lactic acid. Cancer cells can starve a body for months.

Cancer cells switch the pH (acid/alkali balance) in the patient's system and create a positively charged environment in which to grow. Cancer cells have cycles: the pH in the body, normally alkaline, changes to acidic when cancer cells need to nourish themselves to grow. The body's internal environment is changed and the cancer's growth aided.

At the same time, the body's immune system is prevented from functioning because a protective gel is formed around the tumor cells. Cancer cells create specific receptors to attract nutrients and specific carriers to grow and spread within the acidic pH. They connect and attach themselves to normal cells and rob them of their nutrients. Cancer cells also switch electrical impulses within the bloodstream. Cancer cells are positively charged, and red blood cells are negative. Once the cancer cells steal all the nutrients from negatively charged, noncancerous cells, they slough them off and attract more red blood cells.

In the normal body, the pH cycle from 10:00 a.m. to 3:00 p.m. is usually acidic, and from 3:00 to 10:00 p.m., it is alkaline. Then it switches back sometime in between. Cancer therapy must be given when the patient is in the acid phase. Any therapy we give during this specific time will attack the tumor while it is attempting to grow. Nontoxic medications and nourishment for the noncancerous cells are given from 3:00 to 10:00 p.m. while the cancer cells are less active.

Cancer patients especially need to get all their nutrients from the best sources that do not contain any chemicals or preservatives. The goal of using diet as a cancer therapy is to diminish the levels of harmful chemicals and carcinogenic agents that could adversely affect the DNA of the healthy cells, to give support to the cells to get well, and for the immune system to function normally.

Antioxidants Protect Cells from Free Radicals

When humans eat oils and fats, the lipids are rancid, free radicals, or positively charged molecules, are created as the lipids are broken down to peptides and amino acids. Free radicals are positively charged molecules that are missing one electron. When free radicals interact with a cell's DNA, they can change its form and contribute to the development of cancer. Free radicals oxidize cells because of losing their (miselectrical) charges.

The most effective antioxidant to counteract these free radicals is vitamin C. Vitamins E and A are also effective. Other good sources of antioxidants include grape-seed extract, Pycnogenol (a food supplement), and astaxanthin. Astaxanthin is one of the more potent carotenoids because it has specific benefits for human nutrition that far exceeds the benefits of lycopene and beta-carotene. It not only improves the immune system but can also control the deadly "silent inflammation" that can be a precursor to many life-threatening diseases, including cancer.

Negatively charged antioxidants provide the extra electrons to counteract damaging free radicals by neutralizing them and protecting the body's cells. We prescribe vitamins and antioxidants to protect the body from smog, chemicals, and free radicals. These antioxidants are not a cure for cancer but help to protect the cells from further degeneration. Research has shown that by adding only the antioxidant selenium to the diet, tumors shrink from 8 cm to 4 cm. But it is a challenge for patients to be 100 percent cured with diet and supplement alone. They are only one aspect of an individualized program of therapies to deal with cancer.

Why, When and How to Use Fasting

When a patient starts with a cancer program, if he or she is healthy enough, we suggest one to three days of fasting. If the condition of the patient is weaker, then we would suggest only a one-day fast. When a patient is fasting, they are in a weakened but restful state. Their body is supported through intravenous feeding, and fasting gives the body a chance to correct electrical imbalances caused by the presence of cancer.

We suggest people use fasting as a way to correct the internal environment. The metabolic reaction associated with fasting changes the pH level of the blood from acidic to alkaline and prepares the body for successful treatment.

What is a Fast?

Under a doctor's supervision, patients consume only fruit juices and teas while fasting and are allowed to eat fruits only if they feel hungry. This way, patients will continue to have fluids in their stomachs. In patients with cancer, their bodies are in a catabolic phase with the cancer consuming all the nutrients. Some doctors treat cancer by doubling the amount of nutrients given, including proteins, carbohydrates, and lipids. The only problem is these nutrients, instead of helping the patient's healthy cells, go directly to nourish the cancer.

When patients undergo a fasting regimen for one to three days, the cancer cells are unable to obtain enough nutrients, so they begin consuming the body's reserves in muscles and fats. As the pH returns to normal, the level of lactic acid drops in the fasting patient. Once nutrients are reintroduced, the healthy cells and not the cancer cells will benefit the most, and normal metabolism will resume.

In the treatment offered by Dr. Rubio, we remove the lactic acid from the patients during the fasting phase through intravenous infusions (IVs).

Patients are monitored closely. Mineral and potassium levels are increased to strengthen the normal cells in their ability to compete with the cancer. Becoming stronger, the healthy cells will be able to respond better to the therapies that follow. To stay healthy, we recommend a juice fast once a month. While fasting, you must consume eight glasses of water daily to flush the chemicals out of the cells.

After the one—to three-day fast is completed, the patient starts eating again very slowly—first vegetable broth, then broth containing vegetables, and then the prescribed diet we recommend individually according to blood type. With the water that cancer patients drink, we treat it using different filters from Kangen Water to reverse osmosis to be sure the water is free of chlorine and fluoride. Also we recommend filters be used in showerheads to eliminate chlorine.

Juices and Teas

Our cells are typically full of chemicals; we ingest them day by day, month by month, and year by year. To help remove the chemicals and support the body, we use fruit and vegetable juices on an ongoing basis. Juices flush out chemicals that may be attached to the DNA and provide live enzymes to support the good metabolic activity of the cells.

Chemicals are stored everywhere throughout the body systems, and juices and fiber help to eliminate them from the body. We recommend an eight—to twelve-ounce glass of fresh vegetable juice per day, plus an ounce of aloe vera juice. We call this drink a glass of vita (life) juice (made from a combination of two ounces of carrots, two ounces of beets, two ounces of celery, and one-half ounce of cabbage) made from fresh organic vegetables.

Patients can also sip herbal teas, which support absorption and digestion and help to maintain the normal flora in the intestines while helping to freeze tumor growth. Patients can drink different types of teas, we recommend pau d'arco, two cups per day; essiac tea, twice per day; and noni tea, twice per day. Ginger tea, slippery elm, and noni juice are also recommended for nausea and digestion. These teas also speed up metabolic function.

When a patient decides to do therapy to prevent a tumor or stop tumor activity, teas and juices are still not enough to stop the tumor. What they will do is remove excessive chemicals and provide tools to the body so it will function at a higher level.

We suggest patients undergo detoxification therapies (as mentioned in chapter 5) at the same time they manage and correct nutritional eating. This will help to clean out the organs and help patients to become healthy again. This combination of therapies with juices and teas combined with the colonics and enemas cleanses the organs of elimination (colon, liver, kidneys, skin, and lymphatic system) and provides a fresh start.

Recommended Dietary Practices

At Rubio Cancer Center, all meals are served buffet-style. Lunch and dinner have a salad bar with fresh vegetables—a variety of lettuces, carrots, cabbages, beets, jicamas, and avocados—and homemade fresh soups from beans, legumes, vegetables, and vegetable purees. One time each day, we have animal protein for our blood-type-O patients, and once or twice a week, we offer eggs at breakfast. Blood type As and Bs don't need to eat the animal protein. As mentioned earlier, the type Os need a small portion. We do suggest protein as a garnish rather than as the center of the plate. The center of the plate is vegetables, root vegetables, legumes, etc.

The diets and foods served at our center serve as a model for patients to easily duplicate at home. Our staff nutritionist also provides a food plan as well. The body does thrive on variety; some days have a salad with yellow peppers, tomatoes, and beets. On another day, switch up the greens and have carrots, onions, yellow beets, and celery. To help you in making these changes, the popular Whole Foods Market has a Health Starts Here campaign, and their deli and salad preparations made with this label are sugar—and often fat-free. We have health at our fingertips in so many ways.

Nutritional choices are a lifestyle, and the right attitude toward healing your body with proper nutrition is a key. If you haven't been eating organic, now is the time to start.

1) Be sure to use whole foods (i.e., foods in their natural state). Fresh salad, fresh fruit, smoothies made from fresh fruits and veggies, steamed vegetables, and whole grains are all examples to keep your nutrition plant strong.
2) Consume healthy fats, such as avocados, olive oil, and fish oil.
3) Be sure each meal is nutrient dense. If you eat a processed snack food, consume a healthy portion of vegetables with them.
4) Chew your food twenty to thirty times because digestion starts with saliva in the mouth. Chew meats very thoroughly. After consuming meats, proteolysis enzymes should be taken in between meals to help break down the proteins. Patients should never drink water with a meal, but after proteins start digesting in the body, a patient may begin to feel thirsty. Then they may drink water, which will aid metabolism.
5) Some patients don't produce enough digestive enzymes; they don't chew their food correctly, and they don't digest good proteins. As a result, they become intoxicated and poisoned by those same proteins. We suggest taking extra digestive enzymes, especially because proteins must be broken down into amino acids to avoid protein poisoning. Ingesting enzymes combined with the hydrochloric acid already in the stomach will allow the proteins to be broken down into amino acids in the digestive tract. Amino acids will then be absorbed, and with the support of the pancreas, liver, and small intestine, normal cells will get the benefit.
6) Try not to drink water during or after meals because it can stop enzyme activity.
7) Patients are also recommended to consume a good combination of beans and brown rice three times a week. These contain the best combination of complete proteins to benefit the human body.

Vegetarians and Vegans

Persons with A-positive and—negative blood and B-positive and—negative blood don't require animal protein. They can eat it, but they don't need it. Their genes don't require animal protein to produce blood. Patients with A—and B-type blood can obtain all the proteins their bodies require from vegetables and soy hamburgers and steaks (make sure to read labels so the soy has no GMOs). Along with soy products, they can eat beans and rice, which provide the perfect proteins for the body.

Consumption of milk by cancer patients is not good. Since the milk we ingest is cow's milk, the proteins it contains were meant for calves, not for humans. Our digestive systems don't have the proper enzymes to break down the proteins in cow's milk properly. In this instance, the body produces more free radicals, which it can't break down. Instead, we substitute goat, almond, rice, oat, hemp, or GMO-free soy milk for our cancer patients.

Further we recommend that patients use butter made from goat's milk or GMO-free soy. It's easier for the body to digest. The best oils for cooking cancer patients' foods are grapeseed oil, sesame oil, coconut oil, or olive oil. Oils are necessary because the body needs lipids for metabolic reactions in the cells. Watch that the olive oils are pure. If you purchase the cheaper ones, they are often mixed with vegetable oils.

Carbohydrates are required to maintain body weight. We suggest breads baked without wheat. The trend to gluten-free products is prevalent, so a variety of breads made from rice, KAMUT, or oats are available. These breads will provide carbohydrates and energy to the body, help it to maintain weight and provide fiber, and will also remove toxicity from the body. The reason we advocate not eating wheat-containing bread is twofold. Wheat doesn't provide enough nutrition, and it may produce allergies that prevent the body from absorbing nutrients. Wheat contains gluten, which the body may be allergic to.

A lot of doctors talk about avoiding salt during cancer therapy and increasing potassium levels. Many foods contain sodium, and we cannot avoid it. We need it for normal metabolic reactions. The sodium-potassium balance plays an important role in metabolic reactions. In our cancer-therapy diet, the salt our bodies need is introduced through garlic and celery.

Sugar Feeds Cancer

Cancer likes to consume sugars to grow, but the body also needs sugars and carbohydrates for the cells to grow. Cancer cells are nourished by sugars and nutrients that rotate to the right side. As a strategy to starve the tumor and feed the body, we recommend patients consume maple syrup and honeys that rotate to the left side. This gives nutrition and energy to the cells and not to the cancer. If patients are sugar sensitive, then we recommend a no-sugar program. Most people know if they are sugar sensitive because they crave it or when they have it, they want more. For these people, especially avoid syrups and honey; get your sweets from fresh sources (i.e., fruits) exclusively.

In South America and Mexico, the population consumes brown sugar (unbleached), which is also good because it has molasses, which provides nutrients. This way we provide the energy the body needs. For a meal, patients can enjoy vegetables (including celery, corn, carrots, and tomatoes) combined with proteins, such as fish or chicken. But we don't mix the proteins with sugars. We also don't eat proteins with bread. It's too hard for the body to digest simultaneously. All vegetables, fruits, and corn (including tomatoes) are okay. They contain hormone blockers, which help to stop tumor growth. White sugar on the other hand has no nutritional values, and it feeds the cancer cells.

With cancer and healthy patients, we need to eat proteins as proteins alone. If you like to enjoy bread, eat it two hours prior to a main meal. If you like to eat bread with proteins, try substituting corn tortillas instead. Cultures in Mexico and South America combine corn tortillas with proteins. It's a good combination and provides excellent nutrition to the body.

Along with a healthy diet, which will support the immune system, we suggest patients take extra vitamins and minerals to supplement their diet even if it's organically grown food, it may still lack vitamins and minerals. The organic sources of the foods support the body from being exposed to too many chemicals and preservatives.

Vitamins' Role in Preventing and Treating Cancer

Before cancer patients develop tumors, they also develop precancerous cells, often ten to twenty years before the actual cancer appears. We don't know exactly what is happening at that point, but we do know that at the stage when precancerous cells are transforming themselves, vitamins can help return them to normal and prevent a tumor from developing.

A program to change the patient's diet is one of the first steps we use to treat cancer. We use food or food supplements that contain vitamins and minerals to reduce and stop the growth of tumors.

Lifestyle Recommendations

When a patient is undergoing cancer therapy, we must avoid televisions, microwaves, and computers because electricity and radiation can aid cancer growth. Perfumes, makeup, and lipsticks are all full of mercury and aluminum. We suggest patients wear cosmetics based on aloe vera and cactus. We suggest showers with natural soaps and the use of a few drops of lemon juice as a natural deodorant.

All these recommendations, you may say, are difficult to follow, but we need to do it to regain our health. We need to avoid pollution and radiation as much as possible. These simple techniques will help to reduce the level of harmful chemicals in the body and help it to put its entire attention on healing the tumor.

Foods to Avoid

Every day, the foods we eat, the water we drink, and the air we breathe all cause our bodies to contend with millions of chemicals, insecticides, and pesticides circulating through our systems and stored within our cells.

Some cancer-promoting foods such as hot dogs contain the preservative nitrosamine, one of the strongest carcinogens known. Food processors add chemical preservatives to meat because it is very difficult for them to control its degeneration and the bacteria it contains.

There are different foods that will promote cancer growth and others that will defend the body from it. The following foods don't intrinsically cause cancer, it is the sodium nitrate that acts as a carcinogen. The following foods promote cancer growth:

- Bacon
- Hot dogs
- Cold cuts and luncheon meats
- Butter
- Milk
- Cream
- Margarine
- Mayonnaise
- Sugar
- Saccharin

- Coffee
- Alcohol

Substitution Strategy

Because it's a struggle to change the diet, it is helpful to know that we can substitute the foods that promote cancer growth with those that do not. Take the following as examples:

- As a substitute for hot dogs, try soy dogs GMO-free and field roast dogs made from grains.
- Instead of meats like beef or pork, use free-range chicken or shark.
- There are so many milk substitutes to choose from, such as almond, goat, rice and oat milk. The same is true for cheeses.
- Sugar can be substituted with maple syrup, honey, or stevia.
- Substitutes for coffee include herbal coffee like teeccino, green, and herbal teas.

Most humans like to eat a lot of meat and fat. We are not saying that eating broccoli or carrots will stop cancer or that eating a lot of fat will help you to develop cancer, but eating a lot of fat causes the pancreas and liver to overproduce enzymes to break down fat proteins into amino acids. Sometimes, meat contains chemicals, including anabolic growth hormones and antibiotics. Enzymes can't break down or make these chemicals contained in fat or protein into amino acids.

You may also want to limit alcohol because any food we eat that is a sugar or carbohydrates breaks down to alcohol inside the cell, which causes a different type of reaction, an inflammatory type of reaction that can cause a tumor to develop.

Instead, a different type of reaction takes place, an inflammatory type of reaction that can cause a tumor to develop. The chemicals irritate the walls of the colon and may be absorbed into the bloodstream and redeposited in fatty tissue. This is one of the prime causes of colon cancer.

Through laboratory studies, we have found that insecticides, pesticides, and chemicals go to the DNA level in cells, change their genetic code, and promote the development of tumors. By instituting a proper diet based on blood type, we can help the DNA to defend itself by gaining strength, releasing the chemicals attached to it, and healing itself.

Proactive Dietary Information to Prevent Cancer

Some of the foods that defend against cancer include the following:

- Broccoli
- Cauliflower
- Cabbage
- Carrots
- Fruits
- Vegetables
- Tomatoes *Nt shade*
- Ginger
- Garlic
- Fish
- Organic liver
- Chicken
- Flaxseed oil
- Rice
- Beans
- Corn
- Soy

All these foods are high in selenium, which is an antioxidant. They're also high in vitamins A, C, and E.

Extensive research has shown that you can protect your cells' DNA through diet. In investigating the low rates of colon cancer found in Finland, scientists discovered that the Finns ate diets rich in meat and fat but combined them with a lot of foods containing fiber. They found that fiber-containing foods helped absorb and eliminate the chemicals from fat and protein-rich foods.

Ingesting a lot of fiber can help eliminate harmful chemicals from the body. With a diet designed for the cancer patient, we fine-tune the excessive eating of fats. We don't want to allow the body to overproduce hormones caused by eating excessive amounts of chemical-laden foods. An overabundance of hormones can also contribute to the development of breast cancer.

But if we wish to remain healthy, we must avoid these carcinogens and preservatives in our diets. We should use different techniques to preserve and control the bacteria in meat, such as freezing it to keep the enzymes alive. It's a risk most of us are not avoiding completely. That's why we also need extra enzymes, supplements, and antioxidants to remove dangerous chemicals and free radicals from our systems. The best way to eliminate nitrosamines from our systems and support us against carcinogens is to use antioxidants to counteract them, including vitamins A, C, and E and selenium and zinc.

All foods that promote cancer have a delicate effect on one of the most important enzymes we have: catalase, which works with hydrogen peroxide in cell metabolism. Hydrogen peroxide protects cells after a metabolic reaction takes place, but when it is not in harmony with catalase, it can help alter DNA in a cell's genes and cause a tumor to develop.

Since 1961, research has shown that bacteria, fungi, viruses, and parasites invade the body when levels of catalase drop. When this happens, cancer can start growing because any metabolic reaction needs the catalase enzyme to work with hydrogen peroxide to be completed.

We have discovered more than one thousand chemicals in food and water that destroy the catalase–hydrogen peroxide balance. These include sulfur dioxide, sodium nitrate, sodium fluoride, hormones, insecticides, and food colorings. The fluoride used in water causes catalase enzyme levels to drop. Beverages such as cola, coffee, and alcohol are also contributing factors. A study of 233 patients who had developed bladder cancer found that their levels of catalase had dropped, and they had been infected with aflatoxin B, a fungus that infects the grains used in making cola.

Once you have cancer, you are more likely to become better informed about lifestyle choices, such as your diet, that are negatively affecting your overall health. Just as your diet may have harmed you, you can now use it to help heal you.

Some people want to eat healthy but were never given the proper education, tools, or discipline to follow. If this is your case, we also suggest a nutrition-education class, detoxification, or nutrition-based retreat (i.e., health immersion class) to support you as you make this lifestyle change. Some of these locations are available on our *www.breakingthecancercode.com* website.

We do suggest patients get a professional nutritionist, naturopath, iridologist, or doctor to review their dietary needs when the body needs healing like this. See the resource section for some places to search for these professionals. Proactive nutrition is prevention!

Chapter 7

Vitamins' Role in Preventing and Treating Cancer

A program to change the patient's diet is one of the first steps we use to treat cancer. But we don't rely on food alone; we also use food supplements that contain vitamins and minerals to reduce and stop the growth of cancer tumors.

Before cancer patients develop tumors, they also develop precancerous cells, often ten to twenty years before the actual cancer appears. We don't know exactly what is happening at that point, but we do know that at the stage when precancerous cells are transforming themselves, vitamin support can help the cells return to normal and prevent a tumor from developing.

Here are some "cliff notes" on vitamins and how they play a special role in preventing and treating cancer.

Vitamin A

Vitamin A is a fat-soluble vitamin that is stored in fat tissue. In treating cancer patients, we administer it in megadoses because they need ten to twenty times the recommended daily amount. After years of using these high doses, we have found that patients can ingest ten thousand to two hundred thousand units a day without any negative side effects.

The reasons this vitamin is so beneficial are many. Vitamin A protects the catalase enzyme, which helps remove harmful free radicals and protects DNA from carcinogenic chemicals. It is found in livers, green vegetables, and carrots. It prevents carcinogenic agents from attaching themselves to a cell's DNA, which can initiate a chain reaction of breaking the protein and encouraging the development of a tumor. Vitamin A protects cells and helps to reverse the process of cancer-prone cells becoming a tumor.

For prostate cancer patients, we found that when Dr. Rubio added vitamin A to an in vitro laboratory culture in the lab, he witnessed the regression of tumor cells. Dr. Rubio has also seen some cancer cells revert to normal after using vitamin A therapy and concluded that this is a very beneficial cancer treatment.

Vitamin B

Vitamin B is a water-soluble vitamin. It can also be taken in megadoses with no side effects, and more importantly, it works in a similar way to enzymes and coenzymes to facilitate chemical reactions and cell metabolism. Vitamin B2, riboflavin, is the principal B vitamin that supports the carrying of oxygen to cells. There are thousands of factors that influence the production of cancer cells, but when cells get less oxygen, they are under more stress and are more inclined to develop into a tumor.

Vitamin B carries iron, niacin, and pantothenic acid and supports carrying oxygen to the cells. It helps to break the anaerobic cycle of cancer cells and starts to deplete them.

When patients receive cancer vaccinations, chemotherapy, radiation, or surgery, Dr. Rubio's protocol then adds vitamin B2 to their regimen so they will receive better oxygenation and respond better to all the cancer therapies. In some of his earlier research, testing forty-five breast cancer patients after mastectomies, the patients who received megadoses of vitamin B2 showed no metastasis after five years. In terms of the effectiveness, vitamin B2 lasts about nine months from the time it's taken to protect the cells. Other B vitamins are beneficial to the body and have specific functions, but B2 is especially important in dealing with cancer. As far as a food source, liver is the best source of vitamin B2.

The B Vitamins for Digestive Health

B vitamins are essential for digestive health. They are also water soluble. This means you can't store them away in your fat cells to use later; you need to make them a daily part of your diet. B vitamins are mainly involved in getting energy from the food you eat into your cells.

Here are some of the best B vitamins to consider:

- *Folic acid.* Not getting enough of this vitamin has been linked to birth defects. Because of this, many foods are now fortified with folic acid. This B vitamin is especially important for digestive heath because high levels have been shown to lower your risk of colon cancer.
- *Vitamin B1.* This vitamin, also known as thiamine, helps your body change the carbohydrates in your diet into energy for your cells. Thiamine is also important in the regulation of appetite.

Vitamin B2. A shortage of this vitamin, which is also known as riboflavin, can result in sores and a swollen tongue and mouth.

Vitamin B3. Also known as niacin, this vitamin is important for many digestive tract functions, including the breakdown of carbohydrates, fats, and alcohol. Not getting enough niacin can result in a disease known as pellagra, which causes severe vomiting and diarrhea.

Vitamin B6. The other name for this vitamin is pyridoxine. It is very important in helping your digestive system process all the protein you eat.

Biotin. This B vitamin helps your digestive system produce cholesterol and process proteins, carbohydrates, and fatty acids. After proteins are broken down, biotin helps digestive health by getting rid of the waste products.

B vitamins can be added to your diet by eating more whole grains, beans, seafood, eggs, dairy products, and lots of leafy green vegetables. Because studies show that many people do not get enough B vitamins in their diet, a daily multivitamin with B supplements is a good idea.

Vitamin C

Vitamin C is another water-soluble vitamin and has been the subject of extensive research. Vitamin C protects the immune system naturally and makes white blood cells stronger. It works through the bloodstream and creates fibrosis, or the encapsulation of the metastasis of the tumor. Cancer cells are never completely removed from the body. Instead, they become inactive. Vitamin C helps to create this inactivity. It protects the body, prevents metastasis, and works as an antioxidant to remove the dangerous free radicals from the body.

Along with other orthodox therapies, we need to include vitamin C with vitamins A and B in the cancer-treatment protocol. These vitamins will not stop the growth of tumors, but they will work to make the immune system stronger. They work at the same level as oxygen and DNA to combat tumors at the cellular level.

Vitamin C for Digestive Health

Recent research hasn't supported many of the health claims for vitamin C. Although vitamin C may not be as powerful in preventing colds and infections as once thought, it is still important for healthy teeth and gums, which are important for digestive health. Vitamin C is also important for your digestion because it helps you absorb iron. If you include good sources of vitamin C in your diet, you shouldn't need any supplement beyond a daily multivitamin. Here are some good dietary sources of vitamin C:

- Citrus fruits
- Berries
- Tomatoes
- Peppers
- Broccoli
- Fortified cereal
- Rose hips

Vitamin D for Digestive Health

If you live in the northern part of the United States or if you don't get out in the sunshine for at least fifteen minutes every day, you should consider a vitamin D supplement. Studies show that about one billion people worldwide are deficient in vitamin D.

For digestive health, vitamin D helps build strong teeth. The vitamins and other nutrients you get from a balanced diet are essential for your digestive health and will keep your digestive system working smoothly. Many studies show that being low on vitamin D may increase your risk of colon cancer.

Just keep in mind that fortified vitamins added to foods are synthetic vitamin sources. You can get vitamin D into your diet by eating the following foods:

- Fortified cereal
- Fortified milk, eggs, and other dairy products

- Eggs
- Liver
- Salmon and tuna

Minerals

Minerals—including selenium, copper, iodine, and zinc—are found in groundwater. Like vitamins, they also enhance the functioning of the immune system. Because of poor water quality and mineral deficiencies in our food chain, our cells are also mineral deficient and are more susceptible to the DNA changes that cause cancer.

Minerals are elements vital to the human body. We need a minimum of 107 minerals to stay healthy. Some we only need in trace amounts. Some we use as a cancer therapy in megadoses, such as selenium, copper, iodine, and zinc. These are needed by the cancer patient. Also, calcium, magnesium, potassium, and sodium are important. These minerals will support any cell in our body in facilitating metabolic reaction, cell reproduction, and hormone production vital to good health.

As was mentioned before, the tumor removes minerals from healthy cells, which need to be replaced. We also give cancer patients mineral supplements because of the general depletion of mineral levels in our water, food, and soil, which translate to not enough minerals present to support the body in metabolic reactions.

Causes for this mineral deficiency in the water supply and foods are many. Commercial farmers don't rotate their crops as they should. The ground is weaker as a result, and there is too much stress on the soil to provide sufficient minerals. In the 1700s and 1800s, farmers rotated beans, wheat, alfalfa, corn, and other crops, and the soils maintained a healthy balance of minerals.

The use of treated water in irrigation, which contains viruses and bacteria, can infect fruits and vegetables. The treated water doesn't destroy viruses. Excessive chlorine in water used in irrigation changes the molecular structure of the soil, and minerals lose their form and shape, and levels are reduced.

One of the best sources of minerals for our bodies is algae, plants grown in big lakes and the oceans. These support the body with negatively charged electrical impulses in the form of antioxidant substances. Algae sources are good for immediate but not long-term effects in nutrition. We supplement the body with other sources of minerals and vitamins to enhance cell functioning and to support the immune system. Some studies have shown the beneficial effects of mineral therapy. In twenty-five patients with liver cancer, tumor sizes were reduced when we added copper to their diets. In cases of breast and uterine cancer, iodine aided the role of estrogen as a cancer blocker.

Supporting patients with intravenous infusions of minerals as a therapy can further support the body and boost the immune system. This is used in conjunction with lipids and water-soluble vitamins as well as immunotherapy to successfully treat cancer. Using all these methods simultaneously, we have witnessed the instantaneous remission or diminishment of tumors.

Vitamin Chapter
Organic versus Synthetic Sources of Vitamins

Vitamins can be obtained either from synthetic or organic sources. Both work, but synthetic vitamins lose potency when exposed to light, plus they contain preservatives that can affect their interactions with cells. As an example, our bodies need three to five grams of ascorbic acid (vitamin C) each day, which can be obtained by eating an orange. Vitamin C is active in orange peels and juice, but once it comes into contact with oxygen, it then becomes oxidized and loses 50 percent of its efficacy. Synthetic vitamin C only works at about 10 percent the efficiency of an organic source.

Our bodies don't synthesize vitamin C, and we need it as a powerful antioxidant to protect healthy cells. In cancer patients, the pituitary and adrenal glands need vitamin C to keep working. When a tumor has developed, research has shown that patients need vitamin C in these glands to protect their bodies. Vitamin C is also important to keep tumors from spreading. It helps surround cancer cells with fibrosis while they are metastasizing and attaches them to the walls of the circulatory system.

Minerals such as chromium, copper, zinc, and selenium can also be obtained from synthetic sources, but we only benefit 25 percent when compared to organic sources. We can get 100 percent of the organic minerals we need with water taken from lakes with solid rock bottoms. The best noncontaminated mineral sources are ocean-grown algae. These algae are the last part of the food chain that isn't polluted with pesticides and chemicals.

The condition of the soils, which commercial farmers grow food with, has been depleted of most nutrients. Thus fruits and vegetables don't contain as many vitamins and minerals as they did in the past. As a result, we must supplement our diets to stay healthy and turn to organically grown sources for our foods.

Lifestyle Recommendations

When a patient is undergoing cancer therapy, we suggest avoiding extensive and close exposure to televisions, microwaves, and computers because electricity and radiation can aid cancer growth. Perfumes, makeup, and lipsticks can be full of mercury and aluminum. We suggest patients wear cosmetics with an aloe vera base. We also recommend that patients shower with natural soaps and use a few drops of lemon juice as a natural deodorant.

All these recommendations, you may say, are difficult to follow. However, we want to encourage patients to do whatever it takes to regain their health. If you avoid pollution and radiation as much as possible, you will help the body get stronger sooner. There are several devices you can wear or have in your home to protect you from these types of electrical pollutions. These simple techniques will help to reduce the level of harmful chemicals in the body and help it to put its entire attention on healing the tumor.

Chapter 8

Advanced Adjunct and Beneficial Therapies

In our opinion, the best comprehensive approach to treatment includes these adjunct therapies.

We want to offer these beneficial therapies that we frequently use, so this chapter will explain why they are supportive therapies and how these tools further assist the natural healing process. We believe adjunct therapies are the "advanced" cancer therapies because they get the job done without so many destructive side effects.

Our aim is to provide sources that can benefit patients who are in traditional cancer therapy and are looking to integrate some natural solutions. Some seem very simple and are often overlooked. Using them separately or altogether is okay because they are all designed to strengthen the body (and immune system) with the goal of completely eradicating cancer.

Shark Cartilage: A Powerful Weapon Providing Protection

At Rubio Cancer Center, we use a substance called injectable shark cartilage as an adjunctive medicine to our other therapies. The use of shark cartilage contributes to healing but certainly is not the cure-all for cancer sensationalized in the media.

There are three distinct actions the shark cartilage contributes to in cancer therapy.

- Firstly, it activates the immune system as it stimulates macrophages and killer cells (T lymphocytes) into action to help them to recognize and destroy cancer cells. We have studied tumor cells of patients that have undergone shark cartilage therapy and found cell destruction in much greater concentration than in untreated patients. These tumor cells exhibit aberrant mitosis and cellular debris similar to patients who have undergone radiation or chemotherapy. It appears the shark cartilage somehow makes the tumors more susceptible to destruction.

- Secondly, the shark cartilage (as well as other types of cartilage) tends to inhibit the development of new blood vessels to nourish tumors. Studies performed at Harvard University found that calf cartilage inhibited the growth of capillaries in chick embryos. Follow-up studies at MIT as far back as the early 1980s found shark cartilage prevented tumors from inducing blood vessels to grow toward them in studies with rabbits. Medical researchers know that without a greater source of blood, tumors cannot sustain their rapid growth. The cartilage blocks what scientists call tumor angiogenesis factor.

- Thirdly, the shark cartilage contains substances called mucopolysaccharides, which improve wound healing and dramatically speed up recovery. If radiation therapy has been employed, the shark cartilage can also help to reduce inflammation.

Since using shark cartilage in injectable, powder, and capsule forms, we have witnessed tumor reductions on a large scale in a short period. In some cases, tumors in the lungs and those wrapped around major blood vessels have shrunk very rapidly to our amazement.

In different cases of cancer—including bone, liver, prostrate, and lung cancer—we utilize the vaccine in combination with shark cartilage and see a boost or amplified efficacy as the lymphocytes get more active and effective in recognizing and destroying tumor cells. Dramatic changes in tumors have taken place when we've combined low doses of chemotherapy plus shark cartilage and the vaccines.

Hormones and Hormone Blockers

The human body produces hormones in different glands, including the ovaries, adrenals, testicles, thyroid, pituitary, and pineal gland. These hormones maintain all the metabolic reactions on a cellular level to maintain balance and homeostasis in the body. The use of hormone blockers is important because we want to drop the excess levels of hormones so we don't give the tumor anything to stimulate growth. However, we do want to maintain enough hormones to facilitate metabolic reactions on a cellular level.

Tumors grow in the presence of hormones, such as estrogen, progesterone, and testosterone. The presence of these hormones stimulates the rapid growth and proliferation of cellular tumors. Hormones travel in the blood and affect the entire system. Today hormonal therapy can be used with all types of tumors besides prostate, ovarian, breast, and uterine. Hormonal receptors in cancer cells are also discovered in tumors, including blood, brain, lungs, stomach, liver, colon, kidney, and bladder cancers. All respond to hormone blockers, and the tumors stop growing immediately.

This cancer treatment strategy is to block the nutrition and function of the tumor with the utilization of hormone blockers, such as Tamoxifen, Megace, Zoliden, Lupron, and Flutamide. It is important to remember that it is impossible to dissolve or block all the hormonal activity because cellular function requires hormones for living processes. We need specific carriers to block tumoral functioning at the cellular level. At Rubio Cancer Center, our medical approach is to use a combination of hormonal blockers with carriers and oncology medications that are nontoxic.

Hormonal Support for Breast and Prostate Cancer

The most popular cancer for women is breast cancer. To help support breast cancer patients, we utilize Tamoxifen, Zoliden, or Femara. To support prostate cancer patients, we use Flutamide and Lupron. As we utilize hormonal blockers for breast cancer, such as Tamoxifen and Zoliden, they inhibit the spread or metastasis of the tumor. Remember that not all types of cancer of the breast are estrogen positive. Some are estrogen negative, and the prognosis of using these hormone blockers is more favorable in estrogen-positive tumors. When we find tumors in the breasts that are estrogen negative, we use hormone blockers because it's a more aggressive approach and because, at the cellular level, the tumors are using hormones to keep growing.

The use of hormone blockers in combination with a variety of treatment approaches makes a big difference, encapsulating and shrinking tumors more rapidly and successfully. Knowing that the tumor spreads or metastasizes, this is a powerful therapy protocol that we use at the onset of treatment. Keep in mind that the production of estrogen is not only produced by the ovaries but also by the adrenals and pituitary glands.

Using surgery to remove the ovaries as part of a prevention plan for breast cancer survivors or as a preventative measure for those testing positive to BRCA 1 and 2 genetic tests is an extreme approach riddled with some severe side effects, like osteoporosis. This surgical approach is covering only a part of hormone production. The other part is from the adrenal glands, pituitary glands, and fats. From our point of view in breaking the cancer code, this is not a complete solution as its benefits don't outweigh the stress and aging on the body. When we lose too many hormones, we lose muscle mass and advance the possibility of osteoporosis and aging.

By blocking hormones, which the tumor needs to grow, the tumor becomes more vulnerable to destruction by the other therapies. We make specific treatments and use megadoses of hormone blockers for cancers of the pancreas, lung, stomach, and brain. We combine hormone blockers with radiation, chemotherapy, and vaccines and have seen remarkable changes because the patients respond quickly, making it easier to deal with the tumor.

Just like breast cancer for women, for men, the most common cancer is prostate cancer. We have to use hormone blockers because the testicles keep producing testosterone, as do the adrenals, fats, and pituitary glands. When cancer starts growing, we need to block hormones so we drop the levels to a place where patients can make the normal metabolic reactions but not feed the tumors.

Hormonal Therapy Helps Break the Growth Cycle

Decades of studies and research show that tumors need hormones to grow as they need to get all their nutrition and nourishment from hormones. For years we thought this was true with only certain cancers. Cancer and hormones go hand in hand, feeding cancer growth, all in a cycle. The key of hormone blocker therapy is to break the cycle. We use hormone blockers in cycles to stop the tumors from growing and also prevent the tumors from getting nutrients.

As with any therapy, things can change! When normal protocols for breast cancer or prostrate cancer use hormone blockers like Tamoxifen, Flutamide, Zoladex, or Lupron, the patient generally responds well for one or two years. What's happening is cancer cells get adapted, and for the treatment to continue to work, the patients need higher doses. When the blockers don't work anymore, it can open the door for cancer cells to return aggressively. Our approach to working with the hormone blockers is to use them in cycles every month and let the body rest for ten days. This way, the cells won't get an adapted response, and the body will detoxify itself, which affects the immune system and efficiency of hormones.

We have found that mega doses of hormone blockers combined with a low dose of radiation and the vaccines get the tumors to stop growing and help the pain diminish immediately. With the utilization of hormone blockers, we can now use chemotherapy in small dosages.

As stated in chapter 4, we are not too aggressive with chemotherapy as we utilize a microscopic amount (10 percent of the traditional amount) with the application of carriers. This is called IPT (insulin-potentiated therapy) and is especially formulated to transport the chemotherapy directly to the cancer cells only. By introducing the IPT chemotherapy on the cellular level and targeting the chemotherapy to the cancer cells at the cellular level, this helps to avoid the negative secondary side effects. The specific carriers we use are amino acids, insulin, and lipids.

Peptides and Amino Acids as Cancer Therapy

Peptides are pieces of protein that we can use as a cancer therapy to cause the body to create a normal chemical reaction that changes cancer cells into healthy cells.

We recommend the combination of hormonal therapy with peptides, lipids, vaccines, chemotherapy, and radiation in breaking the cancer code for the patient to best respond.

Through numerous blood-analysis and urine-analysis studies over the last twenty years, we noted that cancer patients have below-normal levels of certain amino acids in their blood and urine. These amino acids—specifically glutamine, which helps synthesize many amino acids that you can make within your own cells, and arginine, which few patients produce in sufficient amounts—are key for efficacy in the T cells to increase antitumor activity. These peptides are produced during the rapid catabolic growth phase of the cancer tumor, marked by the large amounts present in the patient's urine and blood.

A new therapy we've developed to use with this condition is, to our advantage, to employ amino acids such as arginine and glutamine and lysine as a therapy. We use peptides and combine these with the arginine, glutamine, and lysine with a specific enzyme. This formula goes to the cancer cells and induces them to begin normal metabolic processes, which starts to diminish growth of the tumor and reduces mitosis of the cancer cells.

This peptide therapy combined with the amino acids affects the cancer cell's DNA and corrects the cell's information in the chromosomes and gives instructions to the cell's amino acids to normalize metabolism. When the cells do reproduce, they reproduce normal healthy cells instead. As the therapy begins to work, the amounts of glutamine and arginine increase in the blood and urine. Used in conjunction with the metabolic program, vaccines, chemotherapy, and radiation, the patients respond easily and quickly, and we've witnessed the cancer tumors shrinking much more rapidly than would be expected.

Interferon Intervention

Interferon, a protein substance that was synthesized by a genetic engineer from *E. coli* bacteria, functions to put a glove around cells to protect them from being infected by viruses. Interferon is produced naturally in our own body by our own cells as well.

In the last twenty years, Dr. Rubio's medical team has been using interferon with success, treating melanomas and leukemia, including chronic CML. Tumors of the brain and lung, liver, and colon cancer have been treated successfully as well. The use of interferon with carriers like zinc and oxygen in combination with the cancer vaccines has been part of our successful treatments. Since interferon was first developed as a cancer treatment, we have used it successfully in clinical trials.

At Rubio Cancer Center, we combine interferon with oxygen and administer it in many different ways. In our procedure, we combine pure oxygen with interferon, zinc, and germanium. Using inhalation therapy, the patients breathe this oxygen mixture three times per day for ten minutes. We utilize only one hundred units of interferon per session for a total of three hundred units per day. Conversely, in a normal hospital setting, patients get five million units per day.

When the patients breathe oxygen combined with interferon, zinc, and germanium, the substances go to the healthy cells and protect the membranes. When cancer cells then try to combine with the membranes of healthy cells and attempt to attach to the genetic code, viruses in the interferon-protected coating stop the action of the cancer cells.

> Interferon stops tumors from attaching to the DNA in healthy cells
> and from stealing the cells' nutrition.

When we breathe oxygen mixed with interferon and zinc, immediately the red blood cells combine with the minerals and release the interferon right at the level of healthy cells. Using this method, there are no side effects. There is no bone marrow depression or any sign of intolerance to the interferon, which are side effects to high doses of interferon. High doses can also weaken the immune system and reduce the number of white blood cells.

Interferon for Lung Cancer

In our immunotherapy protocol for patients with lung cancer, adenocarcinoma, or squamous cell cancer, we use a biopsy or bronchoscopy to get cells from the tumor. We culture the tumor and make the vaccine from the tumor cells and/or the patient's own white blood cells. We use interferon-oxygen therapy when we give the first vaccine. This keeps the immune system very strong and immediately assists the vaccine in attacking the tumors. We stop the tumor from stealing nutrients and see shrinkage of the tumor right away. This therapy, combined with a low dose of radiation, helps us use interferon effectively.

The patient gets the benefits of the low dose of interferon and none of the side effects. With this method, we can use interferon therapy for a longer period of time, and the patients' cells will not adapt to it. In the research that we are doing, the use of this approach has been very promising. We know from the patient reports, lab reports, and CAT scans that this method, having been used over twenty-five years, has been very beneficial. All our lung cancer patients utilize this oxygen therapy while undergoing treatment to ensure the cells are going to heal quickly.

Hormonal Therapy for Bone Cancer

In a patient with bone cancer, either primary or metastasized, the tumor cells go inside of the bones and pull out all the minerals, making them weaker and subject to fractures.

Dr. Rubio's research over many years has involved working with a hormone called calcitonin, a hormone produced by the parathyroid gland. An infusion of this hormone acts as a carrier to put the calcium back inside the bone. It is also an effective treatment for osteoporosis.

With a bone cancer patient, we immediately obtain a piece of the tumor from the bone, make a vaccine, and apply calcitonin hormone every day along with clodronate medication. We combine this therapy with megadoses of calcium, copper, zinc, selenium, and magnesium, which the hormone will carry into the bones. The clodronate medication acts as a carrier for the minerals to the bone cells, resulting in a big molecule of minerals delivered inside the tumor. The cancer cells cannot hold these heavy chains of minerals, and as a result, the DNA of the tumor is broken. This makes the rest of the protocol work faster because you've broken into the tumor's environment, thereby weakening the tumor.

The vaccine, once injected, creates new T cells in the bloodstream. The calcitonin hormone carries the T cells to the bone as well, immediately lessening the pain. With the use of these nontoxic medications and vaccines, we've witnessed bone tumors shrinking significantly.

Beneficial Therapies

Stem Cells

Stem cells have the capacity to develop new cells or rejuvenate existing cells and any kind of organ. They are pluripotent cells in the way they reach out to find what the body needs. Normally, stem cells exist in the human body in small amounts, and these stem cells flow throughout the body, looking for signals of inflammation to fix or repair (i.e., bleedings, failures of organs, and inflammatory processes). They also correct genetic defects and/or boost the efficiency if the number of stem cells isn't viable enough to rejuvenate new cells and organs.

Here is where we get stem cells:

1) Bone marrow
2) Fat
3) Purified blood
4) Teeth
5) Women's menstrual blood
6) Umbilical cord

Right now, stem cells are used to treat illnesses like metabolic diseases; diabetes; high blood pressure; emphysema; lymphatic failure; renal and cardiac failure; muscular atrophy; autoimmune diseases like lupus, Sjögren's, and MS; arthritis; Lou Gehrig's; Parkinson's disease; and congenital diseases.

In lymphomas and leukemia, the first goal in using stem cells is to overall rejuvenate and activate new cells, healing and making the organs vital and functioning as well as putting life back into a balanced homeostasis. In our center, we have the techniques to produce cells specific for the organ that we need. We can produce cells for the bones, brain, heart, pancreas, liver, lungs, intestines, and any other organ of the human body.

We use only autologous adult stem cells, which means from your own body. We can use heterologous stem cells, which means from outside your body, from fats, and we can obtain mesenchymal cells from the patient's own bone marrow they don't have the rejection antigen of histocompatibility.

For many years, bone marrow transplants have been part of advanced cancer treatment. When they do the bone marrow transplant, they are using stem cells. Patients with leukemia and lymphoma benefit most when the chemotherapy aggressively destroys healthy cells; they use bone marrow transplants to build the new cells. The surface of the cells have receptors that either accept or reject the cells (HL2), which means that they come together and regenerate organs and reproduce cartilage, muscle, heart, and pretty much all other organs.

Rife Therapy

As a cancer treatment, Rife therapy works to kill any viruses that may be present within a tumor. Viruses within the cancer cells are implicated as carcinogenic factors that change the DNA of healthy cells to cancer cells. Rife therapy, over the course of time, causes the cells of the tumor to break down, depending on the density and size of the tumor.

Developed by Dr. Royal Raymond Rife of San Diego in the 1930s, the Rife frequency instrument emitted a variable flashing-light source that Dr. Rife found could kill bacteria, viruses, and other microbes. Dr. Rife both identified the microbes and the light-flashing rate (frequency) required to kill them. Dr. Rife further identified microbes associated with fifty-two major diseases, including cancer.

The efficacy of Rife's treatments was verified during test clinical trials on human subjects conducted by the University of Southern California Medical School Special Medical Research Committee in 1934, 1935, and 1937. Dr. Rife had tremendous success with terminal cancer patients in his many years of research trials.

These short treatments were sufficient to kill off microbes within cancer cells and to kill the cancerous tissue itself, one thin layer at a time. This allowed the body's immune system to remove the layer of dead cancer cells before the next treatment. If used at a higher dosage, Rife's treatments would prove to be toxic to the patient, since a large mass of dead tumor cells would be difficult for the body to eliminate all at once.

Rife is a selective treatment on a specific frequency that is aimed at only one particular microbe or virus at a time; there is little damage caused to healthy tissues. A multifaceted approach, as we've discussed throughout this book, is important, however, patients need to be careful not to overload the immune system with too many dead cancer cells at one time.

In breaking the cancer code, Rife frequencies are effective against viruses, bacteria, fungi, or other parasites within the body. When the resonant frequency emitted by the Rife machine enters the atomic mass of the virus, bacteria, fungus, or parasite, it overwhelms it, and it is either deactivated or destroyed. Rife therapy is a wonderful support therapy for a weakened immune system, which is why we've been using it for years.

Rife and Radiation

Rife therapy uses twenty different basic frequencies. Patients undergo twenty—to forty-minute sessions as part of their cancer therapy and as an adjunct to radiation therapy. Many medical professionals use Rife therapy, and patients frequently purchase their own systems. We use Rife therapy in combination with radiation to assist in tumor destruction. Tumors often become adapted to radiation therapy since it is a continuous frequency and it may lose its efficiency. Rife frequencies are intermittent frequencies that don't allow tumors to become adapted to them and can be combined very successfully with radiation therapy. The general frequency of Rife therapy sessions is six times a week, under a doctor's supervision, as part of the detoxification program.

Practitioners need to specifically support their liver against excess toxicity when using all these advanced cancer therapies to kill off tumors or diseases in the body. We suggest that liver functions are checked through dark-field microbiology, blood panels, and ultrasounds. You can also check the liver manually for swelling or discomfort. In the event the liver is enlarged or sore to the touch, we suggest that a liver detoxification program be implemented and that patients refrain from using the Rife technology until the liver-function tests are normal.

Dr. Rife also developed a new type of high-magnification microscope that could observe viruses in live cells and tissue cultures. In his research, Dr. Rife placed a microbe under his microscope while exposing it to a particular frequency that would deactivate it. Dr. Rife painstakingly identified the frequencies, or mortal oscillatory rates, necessary to kill or deactivate hundreds of different types of microbes.

Rife frequencies are not a cure-all, or the silver bullet that cures all diseases. They are a tool that supports and complements all the other therapies we use. The book *The Cancer Cure That Worked* by Barry Lynes details the medical politics that affected the life and work of Dr. Rife and his innovative frequencies and microscopes.

Magnetic Therapy

Magnets have been a controversial means of healing for thousands of years, finally being vindicated with new studies underway in the United States. According to James Livingston, author of *Driving Force: The Natural History of Magnets* and a senior lecturer at the Massachusetts Institute of Technology, magnets were used "to attract diseases out of the body" during the Middle Ages. Magnets are now popular as a means of nontoxic pain control. Professional athletes and lay people alike are claiming magnets have dramatically reduced pain in conditions as diverse as carpal tunnel syndrome, sciatica, and migraines.

A scientific study from Baylor's Institute for Rehabilitation Research showed that strapping small low-intensity magnets to painful areas of the body could relieve chronic joint and muscular pain among postpolio patients. One patient, a priest who had difficulty celebrating Mass since pain prevented him from lifting his left hand, called it a miracle when magnets relieved his pain.

We also find that magnets are an important tool for working on a cellular level to change the cells' electrical polarities. When a patient gets cancer, the tumor cells are intelligent and switch their polarity from negative to positive. Because of the difference in electrical charge, the cancer cells will attempt to steal all the nutrition and oxygen by attracting the negatively charged nutrients for themselves. Once they starve the surrounding tissue and kill it, the cancer cells switch their polarity from positive to negative to reject the positively charged dead cells around them.

Magnet therapy helps us to maintain a negative charge within the body systems at all times and make it impossible for the cancer cells to switch polarities to attract nutrition. This helps us to maintain homeostasis within the body so normal cells can undergo good metabolic and chemical reactions.

Magnets can be applied indirectly to the body as well as directly; they work well when put into the patient's mattress. We align the magnets to be negatively grounded toward the ground and then place small magnets on both sides of the patient's body to complete a therapeutically beneficial electrical field. Sometimes we apply magnets directly to the tumor to change its polarity and use a solution of Ringer's lactate to enhance the electrical charge and assist the elimination of dead cancer cells to prevent poisoning of the body.

Magnets should only be used under the supervision of medical doctors or specialists who are familiar with their effects, as misused, they can adversely affect metabolism.

Electromagnetic Therapies

As has already been explained, cancer changes the body's internal environment from a normal negative charge to a positively charged environment that enhances the cancer's growth while also interrupting and slowing down normal metabolism. In breaking the cancer code, we recommend various electromagnetic therapies that use different types of frequencies to restore electrical balance to the body and normal metabolic processes. Please visit www.breakingthecancercode.com and request the free report on EMF protection. This report will give you details on ionic footbaths to EMF protection devices that we recommend.

Color Therapy

Each particular color has its own frequency and specific electrons. These electrons will affect the human body to change or correct the atoms in each cell to support the immune system and the regeneration of healthy cells.

Interior designers and psychologists already know how colors can affect moods and create physiological changes in the body. White light and full-spectrum light, which mimics sunlight, have been used to help eliminate depression for decades.

Color therapy is another facet to consider when breaking the cancer code. At Rubio Cancer Center, we use a color light therapy machine, which is a simple piece of equipment where patients look directly into a machine. The therapy has light beams flashing through a color wheel. As patients stare into each color for about twenty to thirty seconds, the treatment provides colors from the full spectrum of the rainbow, giving patients whatever color necessary to stimulate the hypothalamus, which regulates the immune system and homeostasis in the body.

Color Benefits

The use of color therapy is an esoteric, experimental tool for healing. We aren't aware of any recent scientifically conducted studies that have proven its efficacy. We have relied solely on reports from our patients and from our own laboratory tests to confirm its positive influence as another way to support patients in breaking the cancer code. Some researchers theorize that color therapy works to either reinforce the positive color emanations or to counteract color emanations from the body that don't enhance health and immunity. The colors themselves are theorized to have beneficial effects on the body.

Red: Red is thought to stimulate the autonomic and circulatory systems. It can stimulate the liver and increase hemoglobin formation. Esoterically, it can represent fear, which steers us in the right direction! It is male (yang) energy.

Orange: Orange is a color that stimulates mental creativity. Esoterically, it represents courage and survival. It is stimulating and represents yang energy.

Yellow: Yellow is thought to stimulate the lymphatic system and enhance the detoxification process. Esoterically, it represents power; think of the power of the sun! Also, it's yang energy.

Green: Green is the life-giving color of renewal, and just as photosynthesis enhances oxygen, green enhances renewal. Metaphysically, it represents the heart and love and yin energy.

Blue: Blue is the color of communication and forward motion. Esoterically, it represents the color of health. It affects the throat chakra and expresses one's truth. It is a soothing color that represents yin energy.

Violet: Violet or indigo is the color that represents intuition. It's a spiritual-activation and renewal color representing yin energy. Churches and religious ceremonies use purple as an accent color. If your cancer healing is a spiritual journey, use this color in your healing sanctuary.

White: The color white can be utilized to stimulate healing in patients with melanoma. It affects the pituitary glands to stop the production of pigment of the skin and helps to shrink melanoma tumors. This color that is worn by doctors and nurses traditionally is a yin calming color.

We recommend color therapy, especially when combined with chemotherapy, radiation, and the immunotherapy protocols. Patients and people in general have different responses to color therapy. Using the color light therapy at the hospital, some patients may feel relaxed or energized following a session; others may feel nauseous or fatigued as the various colors may provoke a sudden healing reaction within the body.

Some patients will feel a need to enhance color in their homes or paint certain rooms during treatment to facilitate healing. Over the years, several patients have set up shrines of healing in their homes and often painted these rooms green or violet to indicate their desire. Once you embark on your healing journey, pay attention to colors that stimulate you and dress or design your life accordingly.

Even if you aren't a cancer patient, caregiver, or survivor, color therapy can boost your immune system and creativity. While doing final editing on this book, Carolyn stayed at a "color therapy" hotel to boost her creative spirit, where the rooms were decorated and painted in neon colors to imitate desert blooms. Amazed at how her health and well-being were affected with royal-purple walls, a neon-green desk, and orange accents, she knew one more time how energizing colors can be. The goal was reached to provide a creative boost, with an endorsement that cancer patients and survivors can benefit from a color therapy room or area in their homes to help them stay healthy.

Chapter 9

Nature Power:
Nontoxic Medications and Herbs

The Greek physician Hippocrates was the first to identify the disease we call cancer; he was also the first to attempt treatment with different natural chemical compounds. One of the hallmarks of the twentieth century was different doctors began using natural compounds to stop cancer. A renaissance started taking place as researchers used chemical compounds taken from the rain forest and other natural sources. The goal was to create nontoxic medications to attempt to control, stop, and eliminate tumors.

As benefits kept coming to light from the use of natural compounds in treating cancer, their efficacy, when combined with traditional techniques such as chemotherapy and radiation, started becoming better known to researchers and medical doctors. More and more studies are showing excellent results and important applications for breaking the cancer code revolving around the use of nontoxic medications for cancer patients now and in the future.

Research has proven natural sources can support patients in stopping the growth of tumors and a cancer's metastasis. These compounds are great examples of physical ways to break the cancer code and becoming more readily available. The following list gives names and descriptions about the medications we have used, with an explanation of how and where they work best.

Nontoxic Medications (in alphabetical order)

Carbatine

Carbatine is a compound specifically effective as a therapeutic agent for liver cancer, according to studies done by Dr. E. D. Danopoulos in Athens, Greece. Researchers believe carbatine blocks the gene 415 in the liver. It also helps to maintain the tumor as a solid mass and prevents metastasis. It is a compound that supports the treatment of skin and liver cancer.

Carcelim

Carcelim is a cream used to treat skin cancers. It is effective against melanoma, carcinoma, and basal cell carcinoma. It contains *Euphorbia peplus*, tea tree oil, salicylic acid, and urea. Following treatment, skin cancers become inflamed, scab over, and eventually fall off, exposing healthy skin below.

Cesium Chloride

When a patient develops a tumor, the pH changes in the body from alkaline to acidic. Cesium chloride works to maintain a normal pH balance, creating an alkaline environment around cells and allowing the immune system to function with normal metabolic reactions. Cesium is an element, a silvery-white metal. The benefits of this element combined with chlorine form cesium chloride. It will keep the pH balance in the body alkaline and assist with detoxification and removal of dead cancer cells from the body.

Clodronate

Clodronate is a medication that supports patients with bone cancer (or metastasis of cancer to the bones) to prevent pathologic fractures. Clodronate, chemically a biophosphonate, works as a carrier to replace calcium in the bones. Clodronate can be used with specific carriers such as calcitonin, a hormone from the parathyroid, or combined with different types of low-dose chemotherapies such as carmustine, cyclophosphamide, doxorubicin, or flourouracil to battle cancer. The benefits of clodronate combined with these compounds help in stopping pain by preventing the need for immunosuppressive narcotics for pain and prevent fractures by strengthening the bones. Current studies have shown that the use of clodronate prevents breast cancer metastasis to the bones.

Coenzyme Q-10

Coenzyme Q-10 is a factor that enhances cellular respiration and supports the mitochondria within the cells to generate energy. Coenzyme Q-10 is a strong antioxidant and removes the free radicals (positively charged particles) that damage cells and promote cancer growth. Coenzyme Q-10's benefits include the absorption of various vitamins, minerals, and amino acids, and the stoppage of the anaerobic cycle, which allows cancer to grow.

Colostrum

Colostrum is a compound made from human mothers' milk sources and has excellent properties as a cancer therapy. Colostrum contains antibodies and proteins that will support the immune system's ability to battle many types of illnesses, principally those of the digestive tract, just as it helps human babies resist diseases. Studies have shown that colostrum stimulates the body to produce cytokines, including interleukin 1 and 6, interferon Y, and lymphokines—all highly effective antiviral substances. It also enhances lymph system functioning. Colostrum's benefits as a nontoxic medication is indicated for cancers of the digestive tract, including pancreas, stomach, esophagus, liver, colon, tongue, and salivary glands.

Germanium

Organic germanium is an element that acts as an oxygen conductor to enrich levels of oxygen in the body at the cellular level. These increased levels of oxygen break the cancer codes by helping the body gain strength to battle the anaerobic growth of cancer cells. Germanium benefits the body to help extract oxygen from food and air and to increase levels of interferon to battle cancer. Since we are dealing with oxygen levels in respiration, a germanium nebulizer is a delivery system that efficiently dispenses germanium into the body systems through the lungs. Germanium is an element chemically labeled Ge, which is found naturally in different plants and fungi.

Glutathione

Glutathione is a compound composed of peptides and amino acids. The primary benefit of glutathione is that it acts as a protection to the body's cells and membranes. It works as a strong antioxidant by removing all the damaging free radicals. Of all the antioxidants—such as vitamin C, grape-seed extract, and lycopene—Glutathione is one of the strongest.

Glycyrrhizin

Extracted from a legume similar to licorice, glycyrrhizin is a substance that is fifty times sweeter than sugar, containing polysaccharides and different oils. When a patient develops liver cancer, we recommend they only ingest sugars to give the liver a rest from ingesting proteins and fats. When combined with the intra-arterial chemotherapy and vaccine made from the liver cells, glycyrrhizin helps to quickly shrink liver tumors. Its benefits include healing ulcers, stimulating the liver to heal, as well as boosting interferon production. We apply glycyrrhizin along with various medications to treat liver cancer and hepatitis.

Hydergine

Hydergine helps to restore connections among the brain cells, resulting in improved coordination, memory, and thinking processes. If radiation has been used on brain tumors, Hydergine is used to help restore function. Hydergine acts to support the production of more serotonin in the brain by stimulating the conductivity of electrical impulses from cell to cell. Hydergine is effective for illnesses such as Alzheimer's and brain cancer. Hydergine is an amino acid derived from a fungus and enhances the effects of a psychoneuroimmunology program, as detailed extensively in chapter 11. Briefly, psychoneuroimmunology is using the mind to direct the body for desired physiological outcomes.

Hydrazine Sulfate

Hydrazine sulfate is a nice substitution for Megace, a medication often used for cancer patients that have lost their appetites and are losing weight. Researchers believe it works by producing a beneficial chemical reaction in the liver that helps to starve the tumor and nourish healthy cells by inhibiting the gluconeogenic enzyme from converting lactate to glucose and feeding the cancer cells. Hydrazine sulfate is an excellent cancer fighter as it strengthens normal cells, makes patients stronger, and allows the body to gain weight.

Immutek

This extract of twenty-eight microorganisms (a culture) found in the mountains of the Soviet Union or the state of Georgia is successful in treating infections of *Candida albicans* and Epstein-Barr virus. Used by long-lived Russians, Immutek helps to normalize white blood cell function, preventing and controlling immunosuppressant (low activity) and autoimmune (hyperactive) reactions of the immune system to make it more efficient.

Isoprinosine

Isoprinosine is an antiviral immune-system stimulant that boosts levels of B cells and enhances T cell activity to battle cancer. This substance, taken regularly, protects the body against viruses, bacteria, radiation, and parasites.

Laetrile

Laetrile is a compound called amygdalin, or vitamin B17. It is a natural agent found in the seeds of apricots and other fruits. It has the effect of producing cyanide, which is selectively deposited in cancer cells, effectively poisoning and destroying them. Laetrile thus acts like a natural form of chemotherapy. It selectively attacks cancer cells only because cancer cells are missing an enzyme, rhodanese, that healthy cells contain, which neutralizes the cyanide. It is not a panacea but helpful when combined with immunotherapy, low doses of radiation, and chemotherapy.

Leukotek

A product that uses extracts of the Brazilian herb pau d'arco, Leukotek has antileukemia properties that normalize blood chemistry. It is derived from bark extract of the red lapacho tree that has been utilized by Brazilian tribes for hundreds of years.

Oncotox

Oncotox is a nontoxic medication that freezes mitosis (cell division) in the cancer cells. Cancer cells are rapidly growing cells. This nontoxic medication freezes the rapid division of the cells and allows time for other therapies to work and destroy the cancer. It acts as a natural chemotherapy, which can be combined with orthodox therapy. Oncotox is beneficial in treating breast, lung, and colon cancer.

Palladium

Palladium is a mineral that can block the growth of cancer DNA by altering the electrical charge within the cancer cells.

Polyerga

Polyerga is a peptide that supports the immune system in stomach and spleen cancers to assist converting cancer cells to healthy cells. It has been used effectively in China and Europe for many years along with various types of chemotherapies. When treating inoperable stomach cancers, we combine the use of vaccines, Polyerga, and colostrums along with a low dose of chemotherapeutic drugs as our treatment protocol.

Selenium

An essential trace mineral, selenium is an important antioxidant that can prevent cellular destruction and assist the body in fending off cancer.

Shark Cartilage

Shark cartilage inhibits angiogenesis, the process by which tumors cause new blood vessels to form to nourish a tumor. It also fights infection, has wound-healing properties, and has antiarthritis benefits as well. Review extensive applications in chapter 8.

Tadenom

An anticancer medication, tadenom, is used to treat prostate cancer.

Thymus Extract

Thymus extract contains different peptides and amino acids that will help stimulate T cells of the immune system to battle cancer, AIDS, and herpes. Thymus extract can be routinely used as a subcutaneous injection along with chemotherapy, radiation, vaccines, and surgery.

Herbs

Alfalfa

Alfalfa (*Medicago sativa*) is used at the Rubio Cancer Center as a general tonic that helps to alkalinize the metabolism and fight cancer. Since it contains betaine, it aids in the digestive process. It is useful to enhance a patient's general energy level, helping to fight fatigue by nourishing the pituitary gland. A helpful tonic for the whole body, it contains vitamins A, B1, B6, B12, C, D, E, and K as well as essential amino acids and minerals.

Other cancer-fighting attributes may be reducing tissue damage caused by radiation therapy and as a fiber assisting in the elimination of carcinogens from the body.

Barley Green

Barley green is a grain from Britain that, through a process of steeping and drying, creates a fermented substance used to produce alcoholic malt liquors. We use barley green to create a process of fermentation within the body that will compete with the tumor for nutrients during the cancer's growth cycle during certain times of the day, as referenced earlier to be 10:00 a.m. to 3:00 p.m. in the circadian rhythm. This competition can help to starve the tumor and encourage the healthy metabolism to gain the upper hand.

Cat's Claw

Cat's claw is a woody vine that grows in the rain forests of Peru and has been used in folk medicines for centuries. Peruvian natives call it *Wilcarra*, meaning "sacred plant." As an herbal medication in use at Rubio Cancer Center, cat's claw contains saccharides and alkaloids that have proven to have immune-stimulating properties along with antibacterial, antiviral, and antifungal effects. Research in many countries since the early 1970s has shown cat's claw's potential in treating cancer, AIDS, allergies, arthritis, and viral infections with its anti-inflammatory properties.

Cayenne

Cayenne (*Capsicum*) is an herbal medication derived from pepper plants. We use cayenne as a carrier to enhance the activities of the other medications and supplements. When used with patients who have developed blood clots, cayenne allows easy restoration of blood flow and can be used in conjunction with the medications heparin and Coumadin. Cayenne is one of the most effective ways to prevent blood clots in patients whose cancer is metastasizing.

Cuachalalate

Cuachalalate is an herbal medication derived from the bark of a Mexican tree. It contains an alkaloid that stimulates the immune system and has antiviral, antibacterial, and antifungal effects. It has very strong anti-inflammatory properties. It can be used in combination with radiation to help stop bleeding when there is an ulceration of the tumor. Chauchalalate can treat stomach ulcers also. It is a formula used exclusively at Rubio Cancer Center.

Herbal Combination Formulas

Cascara ITC Combination: This herbal combination is used primarily to assist cancer patients in the detoxification process. It acts as an intestinal cleanser and laxative, reduces inflammation, cleanses the liver and lymph system, and has a myriad of other benefits. Externally, it aids skin healing and counteracts the effects of radiation. The combination contains a mixture of cascara sagrada, licorice root, rhubarb, senna, ginger root, buckthorn, barberry, calendula, diatomaceous earth, aloe 200x, calcium fluoride 3x, ferrous phosphate 3x, PCl 3x(potassium chloride), NaCl 6x(sodium chloride), NaPh 3x(sodium phosphate) and NaSO 3x(sodium sulphate).

Corn silk KB Combination: This herbal combination treats kidney and bladder dysfunction. It reduces inflammation and pain, helps remove uric acid and kidney stones, reduces bleeding, has antibiotic properties, and helps cleanse the lymph system. Externally, it is used as an antiseptic and aids wound healing. The combination contains corn silk, couch grass, hydrangea, shave grass, cleavers, uvaursi, buchu leaves, juniper berries, marshmallow, queen of the meadow, magnesium phosphate 3x, and nat sulph 3x.

Echinacea EI Combination liquid: This liquid herbal combination strengthens the endocrine and entire glandular system, as well as the immune system. It increases energy and endurance, strengthens the brain and nerves, purifies the blood and the lymph system, and aids metabolism. It protects the healthy cells from radiation, reduces anxiety, and acts as an antibiotic. Externally, it is used to treat skin cancer, warts, and eruptions and aids wound healing. The combination contains American ginseng (panax), Gotu Kola, *Echinacea angustifolia*, saw palmetto berries, sarsaparilla, *Stillingia*, mullein, *Baptisia*, damiana, *Calendula*, anise, and licorice.

Essiac tea: This Indian herbal tea was popularized by a Canadian nurse, Edna Caisse, who has used it successfully to fight cancer. It consists of a combination of the herbs burdock root, *Rumex acetosella*, Ulmur Fuluna, and *Rheum officinale*.

Garlic HBP Combination: This herbal combination is used primarily to treat high blood pressure and blood disorders. It aids circulation, reduces inflammation, helps dissolve cholesterol, aids digestion, strengthens the pulse, relaxes the heart, and reduces nervousness. Externally, it is used to treat ear infections, skin wounds, lice and skin parasites, rashes, and ringworms. The combination contains garlic, uvaursi, parsley leaves, linden flower, black cohosh, barberry, cayenne, calcium phosphate 3x, ferrous phosphate 3x, kali phos 3x, magnesium phosphate 3x, and nat phos 3x.

Hawthorn H Combination: This is another herbal combination that benefits the heart. It treats arteriosclerosis, acting as a vasodilator to aid circulation; reduces irregular heartbeat and palpitations; and normalizes high or low blood pressure. It contains Hawthorn Bark, motherwort, linden flower, Peruvian bark, rosemary, Borage, peppermint, ginger root, *Capsicum*, calcium fluoride 6x, calcium phosphate 3x, and magnesium phosphate 3x.

List of Items Beneficial for Cancer

Acidophilus	Chaparral
Coffee enemas	Essiac
Fito enatogrutinina (from beans)	Flaxseed tea
Ginger tea	Goldenseal
Green cabbage juice	Hyssop
Lemon seeds	Liver juices
Milk thistle	Mushrooms
Noni juice	Oranges
Pau d'arco	Pycnogenol
Red clover tea	Selenium
Slippery elm tea	Spirulina
Taxol (paclitaxel)	Shark liver oil

Chapter 10

Patient Success Stories

> Sometimes life has to turn you upside down
> so you can begin living right side up.

For twenty-five years, Dr. Rubio's team has been facilitating patient healings. A common phrase used when discussing alternative cancer centers located in Mexico is "If they've been in business over ten years, they have to be doing something right!" In this section, we will discuss several success stories to illustrate the power of breaking the cancer code.

Before we start, we'd like to do a disclaimer; sometimes, success stories encourage, and sometimes they don't. We have heard that when patients are struggling and are doing everything right but they still haven't healed, other patients' success stories can deliver some disheartened feelings while listening to or reading these stories. Our first story will actually illustrate exactly this. We will also tell several patient stories of inspiration that were not our patients, but their stories struck the perfect chord to emphasize the methods and mind-sets we use to support patients to heal themselves.

A Battle in the Battlefield of the Mind

A recent patient inquiry with Carolyn began as Kathryn, a forty-four-year-old mother with stage 2 breast cancer, contacted the center. Right at the beginning of the call, the first words out of her mouth were "I'm having a battle in the battlefield of my mind and don't know what to do next." Here is her story in her own words:

"One year ago I was diagnosed with stage 2 breast cancer. Immediately I had three rounds of chemotherapy as my doctors recommended, which shrunk the tumor. The next step was my doctor [not Dr. Rubio] recommended a mastectomy, followed up with radiation.

"Here I am, one year into my battle, trying to get rid of this tumor in my breast, and my greatest struggle begins when I watched a program about an MD who healed a grapefruit-size tumor on her chest, not using traditional methods. The MD claimed her healing was through faith in God, diet, and natural therapies.

"I immediately started on a similar program, using natural methods with enzymatic therapy, diet, and blood chemistry analysis with customized supplements. Ever since my hair grew back from the chemo, so has the tumor! My plea is to find a different way as I have a five-year-old son to live for!

With my devout faith, why is the tumor *not* going away? I've prayed, spoken the word of God, and done everything natural that has been suggested. I am more despondent than ever because I feel like I've failed as a Christian!"

The day Kathryn called, she felt violated by the other MD's healing story.

If her faith in God hadn't healed her (yet) like the faith-filled MD patient's story, it was confusing her, hence the battle in the battlefield of her mind. After explaining our approach to breaking the cancer code, using both natural therapies and traditional protocols (chemotherapy and radiation as well), she had some new insights to move forward with. Her faith was so strong that Carolyn was completely blessed by the call.

> Each person is unique,
> and each story of healing is unique.

She Learned to Trust: Stage 4 Ovarian Cancer

Before we met her, Ginger was told she had cancer, and her doctors recommended a full hysterectomy and radiation. She did the surgery but never followed up with radiation. Her choice was to get proactive with supplements and changing her diet instead. This worked until two years later when she started bleeding and knew something was wrong. Through a series of books and research, she came across Rubio Cancer Center. In a short time, she was packing for Mexico. Here is Ginger's story in her own words:

"Rubio Cancer Center was so different from my other hospital experience. Here, I could feel hope, courage, and a sense that I was going to win! I sat in Dr. Rubio's office, where he looked at my records. I knew I was in the right place when I told Dr. Rubio that together we were going to kill this cancer, and he said with enthusiasm, 'Yes!' Hope and faith were in the house!

"The tumor that I had, caused me to bleed to the point I had to wear adult diapers. An initial examination revealed that the tumor was the size of a small orange. The treatment began immediately. I asked Dr. Rubio how I would know when it was working, and he said when I stopped bleeding. I had been bleeding for months, and it was really beginning to wear on me emotionally. It was within a little over a week and a half that the bleeding began to decrease, and then a short time later, it stopped. Another ultrasound was performed, and the tumor had decreased in size. I left the clinic wearing regular underwear.

"By November of the same year—my initial visit was in April—the tumor was gone, and only a scar remained. One year later, in April of 2011, I returned for my sixth-month visit and am happy to report that it is completely gone! Not even a scar. I would not be honest if I didn't admit that for the first few days at the clinic I questioned everything, and each time my questions, which were really my fears, were answered.

"I will tell you that you have to have faith, faith in the treatments and faith in God. I always have been a relatively positive person, but I learned it takes more than that. I learned to trust. I learned that cancer is just a name, and with each treatment, I would picture the tumor shrinking and dying. This journey has taught me about myself. It has caused me to be more patient, understanding, and not to sweat the little things, and it has taught me to enjoy life. I am so glad that I found Rubio Cancer Center."

Immediate Results: Basal Cell Carcinoma

Jimmy is a well-known and savvy businessman who briefly tells his story:

> "In 2001, I found a skin lesion that I knew wasn't right behind my right ear. Doctors assured me it was no problem, but I just persisted and finally got a biopsy on the lesion. Sure enough, it was early stage 1 basal cell carcinoma. Being in construction in Nashville, I had plenty of exposure to the sun and my lesion led me to Dr. Rubio, even before he had his own center.

> "When I heard about the cancer vaccines, I was immediately impressed. As I patiently waited for my own customized cancer vaccine to be cultured, I did all the health-building protocols recommended by the doctors on staff and thoroughly enjoyed the healing environment and taking a break from my work demands.

> "When Dr. Rubio applied the first vaccine, to my complete amazement, the superficial growth of the tumor on my neck immediately disappeared. It actually fell right off my body, like a scab. I had a 100 percent complete healing and have helped to spread the words, telling hundreds of people about this method of treatment. I still get my annual check-up and find myself feeling at home when I come to Rubio Cancer Center. Over the years, I've sent so many people to Dr. Rubio because I'm so grateful for this approach to health."

Follow the Hope: Stage 4 Mesothelioma Reversed

One day the phone rang, and it's impossible to imagine what you are hearing. How does a young person with a pretty normal life get to be diagnosed with a rare, advanced-stage cancer? From his first calls, we were reminded that cancer doesn't discriminate; it affects people young, old, all ethnic groups, and all forms of lifestyles, from athletes to couch potatoes alike. Here was a call from a young pastor who had a cancer predominantly found in older men, called the coal miners' disease. Here, Kohlbe tells his story:

> "My cancer story starts the same as so many others, but thankfully, it doesn't end the same. I was twenty-nine the first time I heard a doctor speak everyone's worst nightmare, 'You have cancer.' I will

never forget those words. It was those words that set my life on a course I never thought I would be on. Having to look at my wife and two little girls and wonder how much longer I would be there for them was almost more than I could bear. I was in the midst of a nightmare, and I couldn't wake up.

"Being a pastor and strong believer, I had always thought my faith was strong, but this test was almost more than I could handle. I looked to the doctors for support and encouragement but found the opposite. As soon as I was diagnosed, we were encouraged to go to the best doctors, so we went to a famous hospital for cancer in Houston. There, they diagnosed me with stage 4 mesothelioma and told me there was no hope. The cancer had spread too far, and the disease was terminal. At that point, all I had was my faith in God's healing power and a determination to live.

"I had a friend who had stage 4 cancer but was doing better, so I called her up to see what she had done for treatment. She told me she had gone to Mexico to Rubio Cancer Center and that she was in complete remission. I immediately called and spoke with Carolyn Gross, their patient advocate. She encouraged me and gave me the best piece of advice I have received thus far on my cancer journey. She said, 'Follow the hope.' That's exactly what I was looking for, I needed hope!

"One week later, I decided to make my journey to receive treatment in Tijuana, Mexico. I was scared and skeptical, but I had hope. That was three years ago. Today I am in complete remission with no sign of cancer! There is no doubt in my mind that God used Dr. Rubio to destroy cancer in my body, no trace of doubt whatsoever in his methods.

"My heart breaks for those who have to face this disease without Dr. Rubio on their side. His approach is not limited to man-made drugs or procedures; instead, he uses the best weapon ever to fight cancer—my body's own immune system. There is no doubt in my mind that I would not be where I am today without Dr. Rubio and his God-given approach to fighting cancer. Your situation is not hopeless, and I encourage you to follow hope!"

Had to Go to Mexico for Diagnosis . . . Pancreatic Cancer

Mary's condition was like a jigsaw puzzle that finally came into focus when we found her cancer. She has passed through more health challenges than most, and here is her story:

> "At twenty-seven, I started having severe abdominal pain. As the mother of three children, I got concerned when it didn't go away. When I went to the doctor, she wanted to get a CT scan of the abdomen. They accidentally did a scan of the pelvis, so I decided to go to another doctor instead. This time, my symptoms had progressed as I started vomiting blood. The new doctor diagnosed me with a bleeding ulcer and gave me medication that helped but didn't solve the problem. I stayed with him for nearly a year and then started having blackouts.

> "Finally, I decided to go to Mexico to find out what was wrong. Sure enough, when I met with Dr. Rubio, he took each symptom, diagnosed the condition, and by the time we did a CT scan on the abdomen, he found a tumor in the body of the pancreas . . . surely enough, I had cancer. I actually had several complications and finally found out the blackouts were from a swollen ear canal, the vomiting was gastritis, and eventually, a tumor in the body of my pancreas was the obvious source of pain. I had very extensive treatment to get my body back in shape!

> "I've never met such a skilled doctor as Dr. Rubio, and his team clearly saved my life. I talked with patients all the time because my healing journey was a long one and I can help those who are about to give up hope because my life is a miracle today."

Diagnosis is the Beginning of Healing

Judith has a rare form of cancer, multiple myeloma, and a very rare blood disease, cryoglobulinemia, that created a pain-filled existence. She had all her treatment in the United States but is so inspiring to so many with her resilient fighting spirit. It took years for her to get a diagnosis, and 13 doctors, to finally explain certain symptoms. She says, "Diagnosis is the beginning of healing," because for her, it was. She had a two-year process of recovery and was bedridden because of the extent of the disease and the two stem cell transplants she faced.

Today she is living fifteen years beyond what any doctor would have predicted.

So how does she do this? Her self-care equation is impeccable: five hours per day of juicing, colon cleansing, proper diet, medications, walking, prayer, and whatever else makes her life feel happy and complete. For her to show up for life, she does her rituals, having plenty of home time because her immune system is so compromised from years of chemotherapy. She writes books, talks to trusted friends, and does her counseling practice. Her story of commitment to not waiver, get lazy, or be depressed is an off-the-charts success and story of survival. She wrote a book about all the tricks she used to keep her spirit fighting after two years in bed, titled "Elephants in Your Tent," by Judith Larkin Reno, PhD.

Saving Time and Money: Prostate and Lymphatic Cancer

A very vibrant, down-to-earth eighty-year-old pastor was diagnosed with malignant neoblast of prostate and the lymph nodes. When he started to seriously consider treatment with us, we had difficulty fitting into his schedule because of his extremely active life.

Here is Charles's story in his own words:

> "We decided to come to Rubio Cancer Center after my doctor in San Antonio had recommended chemotherapy and radiation. Being in the ministry, when I went to get a second opinion, we contacted a pastor whose wife had stage 4 breast cancer reversed with Dr. Rubio's immunotherapy and comprehensive protocols. Just when I felt encouraged to investigate Rubio Cancer Center, my son had heard about another pastor with a similar condition that had been treated successfully down in Mexico with Dr. Rubio.

> "Obviously, hearing about immunotherapy as a treatment protocol started to sound very intriguing. After six weeks at the hospital, I had my blood levels checked and found 70 percent less active cancer in my body. From these results, I was so encouraged that we decided to have my wife treated for her Epstein-Barr virus through stem cell therapies that was equally successful.

> "We wanted to write this testimony because we are both so grateful that our lives have been saved. We also wanted to acknowledge

that we have in fact saved a great deal of money and time getting our treatment this way."

Plan Your Future and Have Something to Live For

Soaking in mineral waters is always an interesting place to renew tired bodies and meet people looking to do the same. One lovely evening, while soaking in Palm Springs mineral waters, Carolyn ended up talking with three lovely ladies. Eventually, they asked what she did, and she said, "I'm a patient advocate working in the cancer field." One lady lit up as she began to tell her story. Even though she wasn't treated by Dr. Rubio and the team, her story has an important message about a patient's mind-set. Denise was diagnosed with stage 4 uterine cancer. After her hysterectomy, she was getting ready to start on her chemotherapy. Here is what rang so true about her story.

> "I had always wanted a dream house, and my husband was making a good living. I was diagnosed with stage 4 uterine cancer, and just when my body was healing from the surgery, I was getting myself mentally ready to start on chemotherapy and radiation, I found my dream home, and my husband said, 'It's okay if you want to buy it.' So we purchased this home. Almost immediately, my friends began to think I was crazy! They felt certain I was going to die and I was decorating this home to leave to my husband. The reason I wanted to purchase the home was to distract myself from the side effects of treatment. I knew having to meet with contractors daily would completely take my mind off cancer and give me something to live for.
>
> Again, my friends didn't believe me when I explained to them. I love decorating, and this gives me something to live for. It keeps my mind from going negative and keeps me focused on the future with something to do that I'm good at. I cherished decorating and the finishing of our new home in the Rancho Santa Fe area near San Diego, California."

What a success story! Denise healed as she built and decorated her dream home and has been a cancer "thriver" for nearly a decade, enjoying her life, home, and health!

Prayer Relieves and Manages Pain

Prayer is a huge area where patients can make great progress in their healing if they understand the impact and listen carefully to their bodies. Here is the story of a liver cancer patient named Clyde. When Clyde was diagnosed, he was told his was one of the more painful cancers. Of course, who would want to hear these words?

He then prayed to the Lord and asked, "Can I please heal this with your grace and go through this liver cancer treatment without any pain medicine?" He didn't like the way his mind, mood, or emotions responded to these numbing medications. Clyde felt the Lord say to him, "With me and you as a team, you won't need any pain management medicines." Clyde wasn't a patient of Rubio Cancer Center, but his story illustrates how powerful the mind is. He never had any pain medications after praying. We can endure suffering in peace, or we can create suffering in our trials. The mind is powerful—more powerful than we know!

Grateful, He Listened to the "Inner Leading": Metastatic Prostate Cancer

This story exemplifies the power of faith and self-awareness in charting the course of healing. Brooks is a vibrant, self-motivated man who walks his talk. Here is his story:

> "In late October, I had a blood test that showed an elevated PSA level. In November, I had a biopsy of the prostate, which came back positive for cancer. On purpose, I never asked what level or stage of cancer I was diagnosed with. Surgery was scheduled for January. I was not at peace with the surgery nor with my doctor. My wife called one day in early January and asked if I would consider treatment in Mexico—she had gotten a call from a church friend who knew a lady who was treated at a clinic in Tijuana, Mexico. I said, No way.'

> "However, after listening to an 'inner leading' and thinking about the people who offered the suggestion, I said, 'Okay, I will listen to their story.' I spoke with this woman, a patient from Rubio Cancer Center for about thirty minutes. She gave Carolyn's phone number, the patient advocate for Rubio's clinic. I decided—in another day or two—to cancel the prostatectomy surgery and booked travel to

San Diego, California. After deciding to go to the Rubio Cancer Center, I had to deal with some in my family who questioned my decision as well as the doctor who was to perform the surgery. I am a pleaser by nature, and this tested my commitment to me. I had done my research and felt that I was being led by God's hand to this center and treatment.

"When I arrived, the driver picked me up and drove to the Rubio Cancer Center in Tijuana—about sixteen miles from the San Diego airport. That afternoon, Carolyn and I met with Dr. Geronimo Rubio. Dr. Rubio asked me questions, went over my treatment, and told me that he would do his part, but I needed to do my part—to pray to God and to be positive and believe. I came into the clinic loaded with scripture from the Holy Bible, believing that I would be healed, and I had a positive attitude. Dr. Rubio made me feel at ease, comfortable with everything. This helped as my father was a medical doctor—and as a result, I admire doctors!

"From the beginning, I did what I could to get to know other patients, the caregivers, staff, and everyone affiliated with the center—I could feel upon arrival that this is a very special place doing an amazing work. I continue to believe to this day that God, my Heavenly Father, led me to Rubio Cancer Center.

"I believe that I have been completely healed, and today I am healthy and whole. There was a period of time while at the center that I was not feeling well. I went through 'it' in order to get to my healing. My lifestyle has changed significantly, along with my diet and my health supplements and ongoing medications. For me, it was and is so unique that Dr. Geronimo Rubio Sr. and his son Dr. Geronimo Rubio Jr. are on this mission together with Carolyn Gross to help others. Praise God from whom *all* blessings *flow*. I am so thankful that I paid attention to the 'inner leading.'"

What the Mind Perceives, It Will Achieve

In touring her book *Treatable and Beatable: Healing Cancer without Surgery*, Carolyn learned a similar lesson. She had overcome breast cancer while certain that a mastectomy and high doses of chemo and radiation would have destroyed her health. Yet speaking at so many women's conferences and health events, Carolyn heard repeatedly stories of women who requested more aggressive surgery and chemo treatments than their doctor initially prescribed, and guess what? They healed.

These women felt they knew what was best for their bodies as they aligned their minds with traditional treatments and blasted the cancers good-bye. What great examples of breaking the cancer code these patients are, with a different medical approach than we might be offering throughout this book. Hands down, it's the same mental directing of the mind to obliterate cancer, which means success, success, success!

Chapter 11

Self-Care and Psychoneuroimmunology

Cancer and trauma go hand in hand. From the moment a patient is diagnosed, the normal response is shock. Depending upon the diagnosis and the way it is delivered, this will greatly impact the patient's experience. This news can be a blow beyond anything a person has ever experienced before. Health care providers working in this field have to be especially careful in delivering this news and also equipped to deal with the emotional fallout that this disease brings to patients/families.

Optimists can become pessimists. Drama queens can shut down and not express their emotions because they're too scared. Laid-back people, at peace within themselves, can be disoriented, albeit a less dramatic reaction than most. We all have a breaking point, and leave it to cancer to be the mother lode of breaking points.

Breaking the cancer code and making sense of one's life through personal awareness and forgiveness both need to be addressed just as much as medical care and a healthy healing lifestyle. There are lots of surprises that can throw us off and upset us while living with the disease of cancer, having a close family member in treatment, or working with cancer. The opportunities to forgive in life are constant and are important as part of the mandatory self-care needed to survive.

> *If a man happens to find himself,*
> *he has a mansion which he can inhabit with dignity all the days of his life.*
>
> **—James Michener**

Finding and Forgiving

In releasing cancer for good, forgiveness is of primary importance. Dr. Patricia Smith, one of our lead doctors on staff for nearly two decades, reminds patients all the time that they need to heal their hurts in life to successfully heal their cancer. This may seem simple, but it is not easy!

Over her many years of working with patients, Dr. Smith noticed that there seems to be a common theme of deep grief that leads to a negative energy in many cancer patients. This "grief issue" needs to be faced *and* healed. We are not saying that cancer patients are negative; quite the contrary, they are often dynamic, amazingly pleasant, and successful. What we are suggesting is below the surface. While patients are receiving their treatment, it is important to address whatever deep grief and toxic memory as they come up. These experiences have been buried and put away. Now is the time these wounds need to be released. Facing toxic memories is one thing, but healing them is another. Successful healing takes persistence and willingness.

The Power of an Open Ear

In order to forgive, we have to temporarily revisit memories to release them. We suggest patients find those people who they can speak their truth, someone with an open ear, defined as impartial, supportive listeners who won't cast a judgment on you or your situation. When revisiting tough memories, you'll find open ears in support groups, church groups, or therapy environments and with trusted friends and family members. Last but not least, in forgiving, is to call upon your faith in whatever trials one has endured, that they can be realized as necessary for that patient's life path and personal growth.

Rather than living with these past toxic situations as a desperado, find your vibrato. Gain another perspective on the situation so you can capitalize. Don't "awfulize!" We have to find a way out of grief and resentment to make sense of our betrayals and disappointments in life.

As we resolve this inner baggage, we free ourselves. If we can bear the discomfort, we can eventually renew ourselves and find comfort. When we take our losses as lessons, we have the opportunity to integrate them as important textures in the fabrics of our lives. Suddenly we can see our lives with these lessons as the way we're created to be. The resentments, betrayals, and burdens are all part of what make the beautiful tapestries of our lives complete.

Lifelong Anger Can Heal

A very artistic gal named Judi was diagnosed with colon cancer in her early forties. Her doctors gave her six months to live, and she was not a patient at Rubio Cancer Center because we don't give patients an expiration date. Her story is important because it demonstrates that it's never too late to forgive.

Judi frequently "awfulized" about her childhood, saying she was abused by both of her parents. She went through a lot of counseling and was a part of support groups to vent her anger. Most people were repelled by her anger, so her friends tended to all be victims of abuse. Just as she was about to check out of life with this lifelong resentment, one night she had a dream. In her dream (like a vision), she saw that both of *her* parents had been abused by *their* parents. As she was growing up, her parents knew of no other way to raise her. Somehow in the dream, she was able to completely comprehend why they did what they did. In the last week of her life, she forgave her parents. The point of forgiveness is that we free ourselves!

Success, as we've stated earlier, leaves clues. So doesn't it make sense that if patients face these dark phantoms of the soul and forgive them entirely, maybe they won't have to continue to have cancer? We see it in so many patients that cancer can be a vehicle to help them face these difficult situations and forgive. Once they forgive, patients can say, "Cancer was a good experience for me, it changed the way I view life."

Look for those people who you can tell your stories to. Just their listening will guide you to find your own answers in the process. Caregivers of patients need to know that sometimes patients just need to find an open ear. Don't be offended if it's someone else; just let it be!

Self-Care for Cancer Patients: Your Life Depends Upon It

You can call cancer a lot of things, and one reaction might suggest it's a wake-up call to self-care! If you've never had an interest in health before a cancer diagnosis, successful healing patients make health a great interest during treatment and afterward. Suddenly if you want to live, you don't have the option of eating healthy, taking medicines, and doing your detoxification rituals anymore; these things become mandatory because now your life depends upon them.

Diet, attitude, faith, exercise, loving relationships, and detoxification are your best friends in caring for yourself. We've known patients who couldn't follow our orders or their doctors' suggestions, and they lost their remissions. After the alarming news of more cancer, they course corrected and began to eat nutritiously, living like health warriors!

Sarah had a full recovery from breast cancer. A year or more after her complete recovery, she became lax in doing her detoxification rituals and eating the proper diet. These were all part of her home program, which is discussed in chapter 12. The home program protocols are a lifeline. Sarah was a faith-filled woman, very involved in her church and serving others, a much-respected woman indeed. However, her self-care equation wasn't a consistent priority after her recovery. Several years after her treatment, she had a cancer recurrence. We are not saying we know for certain that she wouldn't have had the recurrence. However, if she had eaten right, exercised, and done her detoxification rituals, maybe she would have stayed healthy and lived longer.

Her story is to remind patients that you have the power to choose. If you feel lazy after treatment and your weekly self-care rituals are suddenly offset by all your family responsibilities, you might want to get more motivated. We don't use threat or fear because it only weakens the spirit. We do want to strongly suggest you be proactive and stay one step ahead of the invader, or you'll end up like any battle lost, having to surrender.

You Create Your Own Happiness

Sometimes people don't realize just how much they hold their destiny in the palm of their hands! You can fight your current health scenario and make it misery times miserable, or you can carpe diem—seize the day. Watch out for isolation while recovering because staying connected to people lowers feelings of hostility and depression. You want to watch out for loneliness because scientists have now demonstrated that loneliness has the power to alter DNA transcription in the cells of the immune system.

While recently admitting a brain tumor patient, his wife let us know that their son had recently passed away from a glioblastoma (fast-growing brain tumor) only one year earlier.

Imagine her surprise when the husband gets the same diagnosis. This wise woman then told us she had lung cancer nine years ago and a recurrence four years later. As we looked at her, knowing this family has sure had more than their fair share of cancer, she glibly said, "You create your own happiness." And she meant it because she wasn't glum; she was stalwart and determined.

Stop Giving Your Power Away

Elizabeth was a stage 4 breast cancer patient who didn't have an easy relationship with her mom when she was growing up. From this patient's perspective, her mother dominated Elizabeth's decisions and made the mother's needs consistently more crucial than her daughter's.

When Elizabeth left home, she found herself constantly replacing her mother with people who would play a dominant role in her life. She gave her power over to boyfriends, father or mother figures, bosses, and even religious leaders and teachers at different points in her life. She gave them the role of making *their opinions right* about every facet of *her life*.

Once she finally recognized this pattern, she stopped giving her power away. Her healing commenced when she started practicing better self-care and believing in her power to make her own choices. For the first time in her life, she made her needs more important than the needs of others. In this way, she was able to completely heal and move on to a more fulfilling life after cancer, significantly better than she had before.

Patients need their strength and power to heal. If you had relationships in the past where you gave your power away, now is the time to stop. If you never had self-worth, now is the moment to get it. Patients who have not been strong before and were easily persuaded and influenced by others' opinions, today is your new day. This story illustrates how life changing these realizations can be.

Make a declaration:
Starting today, I will stop giving my power away
because I need *my* power to heal.

Master Your Moods

The immune system doesn't respond well to depression. Since optimists cultivate positive energy, this energy translates to all parts of the body. The same is true of depression. Any negative energy slows down and depresses the activity of the immune system and healing.

Since not everyone can wash their hands of cancer easily, we want to provide you with some tips for mastering your moods when it comes to freeing yourself of the concerns of cancer.

- Stop taking cancer personally. Cancer isn't personal; it just is.
- Watch out; rid yourself of energy drainers and toxic people. Your health depends on it.
- Figure out how to let go of burdens that aren't yours but you carry them anyway.
- Give yourself some new experiences (i.e., museums, art fairs, or Disneyland, anyone?).

Psychoneuroimmunology

Psychoneuroimmunology is a field of medicine that investigates the dynamic connection between emotional attitudes, beliefs, thoughts, and physical health. The study takes into account the interconnectedness of the patient's body, mind, and spirit. It offers a means of psychological treatment for the patient as a whole that provides patients with crucial self-care techniques for breaking the cancer code.

The field of psychoneuroimmunology evolved from the pioneering work of O. Carl Simonton, MD, of the Simonton Cancer Center in California. Dr. Simonton developed an innovative counseling program for cancer patients while working at Travis Air Force Base. The program's central premise was that an individual's beliefs, emotions, attitudes, and lifestyle (as well as trust in their medical treatment) greatly affect their health and ability to heal. In his best-selling book *Getting Well Again*, which sold over two million copies, he documented his work.

Over the past fifty-plus years, interest and research in psychoneuroimmunology have burgeoned. Numerous studies support Dr. Simonton's original hunches by bringing the chemical secrets of mind-and-body interaction to light. In breaking the cancer code, patients need to be encouraged by their doctors to direct their thoughts and emotions to enhance immune functions.

There are CDs provided by experts like Emmet Miller for patients to direct the brain to use visualization processes to place markers on the site of the tumor and destroy it. Mentally, they instruct the immune system to see and recognize the tumors. We've seen firsthand how this modality can boost a patient's confidence in their healing and the ability to activate healing using their minds. We hope to see more of this trend in the future of medicine.

The Brain Is More Than an Organ of Memory

Psychoneuroimmunology takes advantage of the brain's production of important neuropeptides that stimulate the action of the immune system's T cells and directs them to attack the tumor. Our thoughts and emotions affect the levels of sixty different neuropeptides in the brain. Peptides are composed of amino acids, which are the building blocks of proteins. These neuropeptides are chemical messengers that direct levels of activity of the endocrine, immune, and other systems. The brain is not just an organ of memory; it is a powerful organ of activity that can be trained through visualization to create healing images and subsequently create beneficial neuropeptides.

According to researcher Candace Pert, these beneficial neuropeptides use the same receptors on cell sites that viruses use to infect cells. During her interview with Bill Moyers for the television documentary *Healing and the Mind*, she said, "Viruses use these same receptors to enter into a cell, and depending on how much of the natural peptide for that receptor is around, the virus will have an easier or harder time getting into the cell. So our emotional state will affect whether we'll get sick from the same loading dose of a virus. The chemicals that are running our body and our brain are the same chemicals that are involved with our emotions."

Believe: The Power of Belief

We suggest patients pay more attention to their emotions with respect to health. This is true for caregivers and patients alike. Imagine a patient is doing all this great work, directing his mind to destroy the tumor, but his visits with the doctor add stress to the everyday situation. Now, the patient has to visualize his healing and protect his mind from the doubts and fears of the medical experts, significant others, and any other stresses trying to confuse it.

If a doctor inexperienced in immunotherapy casts enough doubt into a patient's mind who is successfully healing, an obvious problem can occur. We learned this power-of-the-mind scenario firsthand with a story that demonstrates the power of perspective.

It's always difficult to watch as other medical experts influence or sway a patient, who is healing, into confusion, but it happens. That is why the title of the book is *Breaking the Cancer Code*. The code involves the mind just as Dr. Candace Pert's research stated.

We had a case of a patient with stage 4 prostate cancer in complete remission that didn't trust he was in remission. Medical professionals at home began to cast doubts into the patient's mind although he was indeed healed. When his hometown doctor did enough tests over two years to finally see a few little spots on an x-ray, the doctor got very excited as he exclaimed, "See, I'm right, you didn't heal. You have C-A-N-C-E-R." This fervor can turn a few hot spots into a full-out terminal problem.

When this patient allowed the medical team to cast doubt and keep poking and prodding him for nearly two years, together the doctor and patient were on a mission to keep looking for cancer. This was a case of the nonbeliever who taught our patient advocate to N-E-V-E-R lose faith in her healing!

> Where attention goes, power flows.

The Creative Visualization Process

This psychoneuroimmunological technique actually sends peptides and neuropeptides from the brain and transfers information to the T cells, directing them to attack and destroy the tumor. Research at the Institute of Psychology at Aarhus University in Denmark in 1990 studied the effects of relaxation and guided imagery on cellular immune function. The study concluded that "even though no major changes in the composition of the major mononuclear subsets could be demonstrated, a significant increase in natural killer cell function was demonstrated. This data suggests that relaxation and guided imagery might have a beneficial effect on the immune defense and could form the basis of further studies on psychological intervention and immunological status."

We recommend, as part of self-care, that patients use active visualization as part of their program. Before beginning the process, the patient must be totally relaxed. We instruct them to breathe in and out deeply and slowly twenty times and to visualize the number as the count decreases from 20 to 1. Each number is a more relaxed level of visualization. As they say the number 20, they breathe deeply, relaxing muscles and tension, then the number 19 while breathing deeply and relaxing even more, and so on down to 1.

Once the patient is relaxed, we then instruct them to use their imagination to visualize the cancer being destroyed. Play a movie in their minds where some strong warrior—spacemen, army tanks or a spaceship, Jesus, an archangel, white light, Pac-Man, a great white shark, or whatever they imagine best—goes to the affected organ or tumor and assists the T cells to attack and destroy it.

Creative Visualization

Patients must believe in the therapies for them to effectively heal their bodies. All the current therapies, surgeries, chemotherapies, radiations, vitamins, vaccines, and others work more effectively when the patient believes that they will work. Psychoneuroimmunology enhances the efficacy of all the other therapies, and we use it to treat our cancer patients. When psychoneuroimmunology is used, the pain stops quickly, the tumor shrinks rapidly, and the immune system functions more effectively.

An experiential part of using the mind to kill cancer is asking patients to draw pictures that illustrate how the immune system is working in their bodies or how their bodies are killing the invader cells. This is often an enjoyable experience even for less artistic people because it expresses how they feel about their therapies. We ask them to draw pictures of their tumors decreasing in size or illustrate the pain/discomfort being eliminated from their bodies.

The drawings can reveal a lot, as patients will respond if they can clear their emotional states. As an example, some patients use black colors and draw caskets when asked to create a picture of the immune system. This indicates that the patient is thinking subconsciously that he or she will die. Others draw with blue and green colors and make pictures with a lot of water, waves, swimming pools, or showers. These drawings indicate that they are thinking of healing their bodies.

Using another technique, we ask patients to list on paper all the things they don't like in their lives and then toss the paper out. This process helps the patient release a lot of negative emotions due to what aren't working for them in their lives. An additional technique is self-talk in the mirror, where the patient looks directly into their own eyes to affirm their own perfect health and wholeness. Some patients feel empowered by commanding the cancer to leave because it's not welcomed.

Every individual is different and has a different perspective of life. These techniques will support patients in using their brainpower to heal themselves. Changing a patient's attitude about cancer is the most important thing we do to help them heal. We try to eliminate some of cancer's frightening stigma by labeling it "the invader" instead.

We like to emphasize continually to a patient that cancer does not have to be the end of a life, but instead, it can the beginning of a new life. We use the tools of psychoneuroimmunology to help them to begin this new life in their bodies.

Laugh Yourself Well

Other recent research links laughter with many positive effects within the body. Laughter not only reduces the level of stress-induced hormones; it also increases natural-killer-cell activity in the immune system that is so vital to fighting and preventing diseases such as cancer. Give yourself or your patient the gift of collecting a series of humorous DVDs so you can take advantage of the healing power of laughter. In the future, a prescription of comedy movies may prove to help patients laugh their cancers away!

We want to strongly emphasize that the role of neuropeptides in regulating the immune system has far-reaching consequences for medicinal practices. As the mind-and-body link is now proven in the laboratory, the resulting implication that emotions and attitudes can enhance healing and prevent diseases is changing the future of medicine.

Stay Calm and Carry On . . . Self-Care and Carry On

The slogan "Stay calm and carry on" was popular during WWII, and it was Winston Churchill's advice to his people. We want to mention that our approach is "Self-care and carry on" and live as normal a life as possible. This is important not only during treatment but after as well. By carrying on with life like it is normal, this tricks your mind into thinking all is well. However, carrying on with work, family, or social obligations when you aren't at full strength isn't good. You do want all your energy to get well, so life balance is essential and necessary.

When you are staying calm and carrying on, you want to protect yourself during times that are sometimes hectic. Early winter, when flus and colds are going around or when you hit a holiday season, be sure to protect yourself. Friends are good medicines, family too, so have your visits and gatherings; just be cautious so you don't deplete yourself. You have to be aware of your immune system now, and you may not be able to fight off the colds and flus that friends can bring. Now is the time to know your limits and adhere to them.

So how do patients, caregivers, and healthcare providers make self-care a priority when life-and-death matters can be at stake? Since our survival is a natural, instinctive process, we have to listen carefully to know when our tanks are too low to do more. With the swirling chaos of cancer, we still need to be reminded that our own health matters even when we're deeply involved and committed to helping others.

Now that we have reviewed self-care for patients in step-by-step detail, here are a few more suggestions for family members and caregivers assisting patients and the medical professionals involved in helping those touched by cancer.

Self-Care: Family Members and Caregivers

How wonderful that you have given your time, love, and energy to help patients heal. However, do you know the signs of burnout and fatigue? Are you getting some downtime for yourself so you can continue to support your loved ones?

Guess what, you have to in order to stay sane, helpful, and healthy. The good news for you is you can exercise, socialize, and regroup more easily since you have your health. Cancer isn't invading your body, and your mind can make better assessments and decisions. But don't underestimate what this stress is doing to you; restless or interrupted sleep and ignoring your health strategies can deplete you physically as much as the disease.

Here are a few ideas for your self-care regimen list:

- Go outside and get fresh air.
- Take walks and exercise regularly.
- Watch comedies.
- Call trusted, supportive friends.

- Get time off from caregiving to participate in activities that give you joy (i.e., church, concerts, sports, a favorite restaurant). Just change your scenery up so you don't get depressed.

As a caregiver, you have at least two important goals: alleviate stress and keep your spirits up. You are the life source and sometimes life force that keeps the patient alive. So whatever it takes to keep you going is important. You also need to be rewarded for your heroic efforts here. Give yourself a gift or joy reminder; this can be a plant or a piece of jewelry. Just something visual that says . . .

Beauty abounds. Life is not cancer!

Self-Care for Caregivers

Love and caring are often what really heal patients, so caregivers can feel deeply obliged to be available and make their loved one the center of the universe. However, when the road to recovery is months or years, caregiver burnout is a pit of despair you want to avoid. Giving yourself breaks and time to enjoy life is imperative. Start sooner than later to allow yourself time off to keep yourself in balance.

Some people are so fulfilled in the caregiver role that this isn't as imperative. However, you have to self-monitor constantly so you don't end up resentful, lashing out your unmet needs onto someone who is battling for their life.

Self-Care for Health Practitioners and Medical Providers

What a heroic task you were chosen for to do to earn a living. We've often heard that there are no cruel people who do hospice work. Well, we can hope the same is true for the doctors and nurses who provide healing for cancer patients. When you deliver bad news to your patient, this blow can be beyond anything this person has ever experienced before. Health care providers working in this field have to be specially equipped to deal with the emotional fallout that this disease brings.

With this chosen profession, we have to be able to do the work and let it go! This takes years for most health providers. It is imperative that the art of detachment is learned so health providers can find meaning in their own lives, or they will burn out. Practitioners can't give nourishment to others if their own houses aren't in order. To facilitate healing and give hope to those in need, be strong as you find hope and humor within all the perplexities in the trials of human life.

One of Dr. Rubio's early lessons happened when he was administering his precise treatment and the patient wasn't responding. He kept worrying and worrying on why wasn't this patient responding, and he'd think about the case in his off hours. Then someone sat him down and said, "Your job is to provide the very best medical care, and the rest is out of your hands." When a doctor plays the heroic role of saving lives, they still aren't God. Life has a way of teaching us all about the human condition and our vulnerability at certain times. Those who are exalted will be humbled, and those who are humbled will be exalted. Does this sound like a never-ending cycle of balance? To us it does.

Trying to find balance in her role as a patient advocate, Carolyn found she sometimes learns best from other people's stories. She reached out to Sandra, a thirty-year nursing veteran, to gain a perspective on this. Sandra told her a profound story about a priest who was serving his congregation wholeheartedly, and for all his hard work, he was given the reward of a year's sabbatical. That's right, time off for good behavior! For the priest, this time off turned out to be the hardest year of his life.

What he found out was, his whole reason for being was completely entrenched in giving to others. When it came time for his own *self-renewal*, he was desolate and depressed. He couldn't stand to be alone with himself because he felt that if he wasn't serving, he wasn't living. As Sandra told this tale to Carolyn, she was trying to detach from some tough client cases and find some peace in her own alone time. How many health care professionals have felt this same way?

Especially in healthcare, no matter what your chosen profession is, life has to be balanced so we can give to ourselves and our families when we are done giving to others. If we lose this giving-to-ourselves piece, we must find ways to correct it and safeguard from burnout.

Just as patients, caregivers, and medical professionals all need to practice self-care, we have to all work with our minds in creating and sustaining health. As stated earlier, *the doctors can only provide the medicine.* Next comes the patients' and caregivers' work to keep a healing consciousness to allow health to be restored.

In breaking the cancer code, you want to invest energy to create a healing environment and envision your patient's cancer leaving the body. Use the mind to empower the immune system to be strong and virile. This psychology that thoughts are things actually has an impact and imparts the message to the patient's body.

Getting Yourself Ready

Patients must truly believe in all the therapies, procedures, and medications for them to be effective and helpful. If you reject the therapy, your body will not respond as effectively. This is why some people vomit even before they receive chemotherapy or radiation; it's the memories in their brains causing them to respond adversely. We constantly reinforce to our patients that they must believe the therapies will heal their bodies and not hurt them. This is why psychoneuroimmunology and self care are so powerful and effective in the healing process.

Chapter 12

Patient Prevention Power

Patient Power

Once you're healed, it is imperative to direct your mind and power to continued health and healing. This is a profound and worthwhile process. When the work of forgiveness is done, direct your endeavors to maintaining your health and exploring the boundaries of what support you need to stay in good stead. You have to know your limits and exert your power so you don't overdo and create the problem of too much stress or overload. We want you to know that it is completely possible to break the cancer code with a lifestyle of self-care and prevention.

> Every second, every minute, every day, every hour,
> the key to successful healing is to claim your patient power.

It's What You Do with What You Have

As always, the initial treatment methods discussed throughout this book began with one amazing patient that trusted immunotherapy and Dr. Rubio to break the cancer code. This story is so significant that we wanted patients to know that prevention strategies can be a new beginning. This is the story of a twenty-five-year-old brain tumor survivor who likes to say, "I have a lot to thank cancer for!"

Dan Drost is the embodiment of patient power. He was one of Dr. Rubio's first patients, and his healing story is told in his book titled *A Choice to Live*. When Dan was initially diagnosed in 1987, he was given three months to live by his Canadian medical doctors because of his rapidly growing glioblastoma, a brain tumor. That death sentence didn't stop Dan from using his patient power to recover and using his life as an instrument to serve others. He is one impressive man, and his story exemplifies prevention, which is meeting each and every obstacle, no matter how difficult, with hope and healing.

Diagnosis: Glioblastoma (brain tumor)

Dan's symptoms started in 1987, when he suffered with severe cerebral edema (brain swelling) that caused him to experience headaches, profuse vomiting and partial leg paralysis. He underwent a CAT scan in Canada, which revealed a large brain tumor and his Canadian doctors confirmed the diagnosis as glioblastoma.

Upon arrival at Dr. Rubio's Cancer Center, the doctor's first priority was to stop the edema and then stop the tumor from growing. He administered a specific antiedema medication, mannitol (a diuretic), and a low dose of the antisteroid dexamethasone to diminish the edema of the brain and stop the vomiting.

When the medications began to take effect, Dan became more coherent. At this point, Dr. Rubio went into great detail to outline his methods of using the patient's own immune system to reverse cancer and develop customized vaccines. Because of the edema, there was no way to get a piece of the tumor, and surgery was ruled out. Instead, his blood and urine were collected, and Dr. Rubio used the antigens to make the vaccines.

Additionally, Dr. Rubio administered a low dose of radiation (only 1,000 rads) solely for the purpose of encapsulating the tumor. In conjunction with the radiation, detoxification techniques were used to remove radiation from the body, such as EDTA chelation, green cabbage poultices, green cabbage juice, and baths with baking soda, ginger, and salt.

After twenty-one days of employing these therapies, the edema diminished, the tumor began to shrink and the headaches and vomiting stopped. Dan was able to walk normally again and mental state returned to normal. He was discharged from Dr. Rubio's hospital after five weeks. Three months later, an MRI showed the tumor had shrunk 80 percent. Slowly but surely, over a course of several years, Dan diminished his immunotherapy vaccines and extensive treatment. For over twenty years, his quality of life has been good!

A conversation with Dan is always a delight for our patients and staff. His example and fighting spirit make him an inspiration and healing influence to internationally known business tycoons and celebrities as well. If someone thinks they are having tough times, Dan has persevered through more challenges than most will ever know! His method of helping people navigate challenges and trials is remarkable because he *owns the space of one who knows*. He espouses wisdom like "Focus on your strengths, and your weaknesses will take care of themselves." Dan's core message is always "It's not what you have, it's what you do with what you have!" His book is listed in the resource section.

Dr. Rubio's Notes on Brain Cancer

It is difficult to perform a biopsy on a brain tumor patient because of the edema. Instead, we use a CAT scan to locate the tumor. A needle or spinal fluid tap is used to obtain telltale tumor-marking materials. We can obtain tumor cells from the urine and antigens from the blood. The patient starts with radiation therapy along with vaccines and the metabolic program. Radiation is used only in low doses to immediately encapsulate the tumor and not damage the healthy cells.

In traditional medicine, patients usually go through surgery when doctors find brain cancer. Unfortunately, brain cancer cells go deeply into the brain. If patients decide to undergo brain surgery, they need to know that surgeons are never able to eliminate all cancer with one operation. They may also suffer side effects from the lesions of the surgeries.

The Number One Rule—Think Health, Not Cancer!

Esther Palomino is a determined woman who worked very hard to regain her health. She has had no tumor activity in fourteen years and feels normal again. Remembering how frightened and stressed she was when we had our first conversations, we told her that the rule no. 1 was to not think anymore about cancer! Now is the time for her to start healing and begin thinking about health. We used techniques of psychoneuroimmunology, and she responded very nicely. As of today, her immune system is able to keep her cancer under control, and she has no tumor activity.

Watching people with stage 4 cancer stay positive and resilient during their treatments is always inspirational. The earlier chapters devoted to self-care and psychoneuroimmunology lead the way for the always important patient power mind-set. In breaking the cancer code, the lifestyle and directing the mind to healing are still, to this day, the patient's job.

Carolyn met a woman who had traditional treatment for breast cancer, and she said, "I don't do any of that pink ribbon stuff, I don't even want to think about cancer." She has been cancer-free for five years. So whatever method you use to master your moods, it is paramount in the healing process.

Patients Help Each Other Heal

John, a sixty-year-old glioblastoma patient arrived at the center with impaired motor skils. He had become completely dependent upon his wife to dress, bathe, and care for him. His speech centers were not affected, so he could speak well, but his rationale and mood were violent and abrupt. When he arrived at the hospital, he arrived with a negative attitude and didn't hold back. No one on staff had to guess what John was feeling. Two weeks before John was admitted, Tito, another patient with glioblastoma, had arrived. Personality-wise, he was the opposite of John; Tito was mild mannered.

Tito was shy and didn't speak much and kept to himself as though he wanted to be isolated from everyone. Having these two patients with similar conditions yet completely opposite personalities was interesting to watch. As Tito healed, this quiet and shy man became much more social as his tumor shrunk. He started to take quite an interest in John as he came on board and instantly became John's patient coach and number one encourager.

There was an ongoing exchange, and the result was noteworthy. John, who was normally a bit abrupt, softened as his tumor healed, and he was so touched by his partnering with Tito that they brought out the best in each other. This demonstrates a whole new perspective and bonus to patient power. An offshoot of treatment is a new approach to life that is enriching for patients who face their challenges valiantly. We see this repeatedly and wish to impart the hope that happens as people heal the infirmity of cancer together while healing their lives.

There Is No Imperfection in Perfection

Joulietta arrived, and you knew right away this lady had a certain flair!

She worked in the European world of entertainment. She was a promoter and knew how to take great talents and promote their careers. Glamour was a big part of her world.

On the backdrop of her life, beauty production and talent were her canvases. Inside this Farrah Fawcett–like beauty was metastatic colon cancer that had traveled to her liver.

When her healing began, she was so confident that she would succeed quickly. Cancer didn't belong in her body, and she was going to get rid of it fast or, at least, with certainty. As part of her preparation, we tested cancer cells to make sure they were responding to chemotherapy. With this chemo-sensitivity test, it was Gemzar that was needed to be given. Knowing that Gemzar causes hair loss, which would impact Julian's image, we went to work preparing her for this change.

That news wasn't welcomed, as her flowing long hair, a thick ensconce of highlights and lowlights, was her crowning touch. Her hair was its own work of art. One morning she woke up and started to pull it out, clump by clump. Soon the pile of hair was a foot high.

Each clump brought more tears. She felt like all her beauty was being pulled out of her that morning and there was nothing left to fight for. Of course, this was a moment of temporary insanity that needed help. In the midst of this terrible loss, the call of the day was to shift the situation from victim to victor. We asked her to affirm with each hair clump pulled out that she is ready now for a more beautiful life after this cancer is gone. She had faith that God created a perfect world, and when she focused her mind on thoughts of perfection, then everything else went away. Just this simple act of validating perfection in the imperfection can invalidate the negativity, fear, and gloom of any disease.

Prayer Is Prevention Power

Carolyn met Tony after a blues concert. Her friend Jim Gibson was playing with the Mighty Mo, and she went to enjoy their music. After this concert of great blues and inspiration, she met the band, and Jim talked about her work with cancer patients. This got the attention of a drummer who had survived lung cancer four times.

He approached her to tell his cancer story, more specifically his healing story and how he finally got free of lung cancer. He had a silver-dollar-sized tumor in his lungs when he started his last treatment where he was accepted in a trial for a new medication. His grandmother was a very religious woman and was praying daily for her grandson's life. Each week, his grandmother prayed over olive oil and told him during his treatment to drink one teaspoon of the oil each day. He thought she was a little crazy with this, so he put the oil on a shelf in a cupboard. One day she asked how he was doing because the treatment wasn't making a substantial difference. She said to him, "You're not drinking my oil, are you?" Of course, she was right, and he felt ashamed. At that point, he had an 8-cm tumor in his lungs. He drank the oil each day as she instructed, and the tumor was gone in ten weeks.

Here's to the power of faith and lifestyle changes. When he got a clean bill of health after the olive oil healing, he has been free of cancer ever since. His patient power is having a positive attitude, being a loving father, drinking fresh juices daily, exercising regularly, and making the most of life.

Happy Living Is Medicine

Brenda is another great story of resiliency and positivity when you have a cancer diagnosis. She was diagnosed with stage 4 breast cancer and didn't have any surgery because she just didn't feel it was necessary. Talk about being a nonconformist! She works at a glorious hot springs spa in South California, and she has done a minimal amount of treatment. She's had hormone-blocker medicines and lives a healthy life at a mineral springs spa, where she partakes of mineral waters often. She loves her husband, loves her work, and is involved in making the world a better place. Her tumor markers continue to go down as she keeps on monitoring her constantly improving condition. She really hasn't done anything dramatic to heal cancer; she just keeps living a lifestyle of cancer prevention rather than cancer treatment.

Prevention Power

We want to equip you with some prevention strategies as well as the home program we give to patients at Rubio Cancer Center. We encourage any cancer survivor to have the ultimate patient-power prevention strategy to win their war on cancer. To demonstrate how we address cancer prevention, let's begin with the ten golden rules of health, and hopefully, you can get a few glimpses on where and how to strengthen your approach to ultimate health success.

Ten Golden Rules of Health

1. Stop putting poisons into your body (i.e., artificial sweeteners, hormones, preservatives, pesticides, nicotine, alcohol).
2. It takes five to seven times the normal amount of nutrition to rebuild and repair than it does to maintain health.
3. Be *patient!* Nothing heals in the human body in less than three months. Add to that one month for every year that you have been sick.
4. Have moderation in all things.
5. Make time for peaceful reflection in nature.
6. Live closer to God.
7. *You* must take responsibility for your life.
8. Eat as much raw food as possible.
9. Exercise regularly for the rest of your life.
10. Practice and learn to understand completely Hering's law of cure, which is "All cure starts from within and from the head down in reverse order as the symptoms have appeared."

Beware, you can be killed or cured from the kitchen table.
Your knife, fork, and spoon
can be the most dangerous weapons you ever put in your hands.

Reduce Your Risk Factors—Diet Is Number One

Here is an example of the Rubio Cancer Center Home Program that we recommend for our patients. Diet is of utmost importance to prevent and overcome disease. If you had a bad diet before and are cured of cancer and then go back to a bad diet, guess what will happen again? This home program is what is given to help support your immune system and to help you have a healthy, long life. The better you attend to your diet, the less need you will have for supplements in restoring your body back to health.

Home Program Recommendations

Diet and Food:

1. No junk food, especially while in treatment!
2. Don't use aluminum pans or skillets. The aluminum leeches into the food during cooking, and aluminum poisoning is always somewhat involved with Alzheimer's disease.
3. Use stainless steel, waterless, glass, or ceramic pans and skillets for cooking.
4. Limit the use of a microwave oven. Microwave ovens change the molecular structure of food and release radiation while being used. Standing in front of a microwave in use can cause cataract, glaucoma, and cancer. Microwaves can be used for heating water.
5. Avoid the use of fluoride toothpaste. Fluoride is a poison that can cause periodontal diseases. Fluoride is the residue left over from making atomic bombs, aluminum, and fertilizers. Use a more natural toothpaste.
6. Never use food enhancers, such as monosodium glutamate, as this type of seasoning preserves food but can cause cancer and allergenic shock.
7. Avoid artificial sweeteners and white sugar. Saccharin causes cancer while aspartame can cause brain damage and other problems.
8. Best to eat romaine, butter leaf lettuce, and green or red lettuce. Buy organic produce! If you don't, always wash your fruits and vegetables with a natural vegetable-oil soap to remove pesticides. Limit iceberg lettuce; it can be an irritant to bowels and cause water retention.
9. Preferred methods of cooking are to boil, bake, or steam. Here are some helpful statistics: 120 degrees of heat destroys enzymes, 180 degrees destroys minerals. Vitamins are destroyed somewhere in between. Rarely eat fried or barbequed food. The effect of eating barbequed meat is like smoking cigarettes. Cigarettes are a known carcinogen and have over forty different poisons in them.
10. You should eat brown rice and beans served together three times per week. With this, eat lots of oranges and yellow foods. Eat as much raw food as possible. Eat fruits thirty minutes before meals or in between meals as a snack or as a meal itself. Do not eat fruits with meals because fruits are 95 percent distilled water, which dilutes down your digestive juices, causing digestive problems resulting in bloating and gas.
11. One of the major deficiencies in sick people is an HCl deficiency. A small baby does not start to develop HCl until about six months

of age. This is why we should not start a baby on solids until then. HCl breaks down all solid foods and fibers that hold foods together. Vegetables do have fibers. We cannot absorb out nutrients unless they have been turned into a liquid called chyme. Solids released from the stomach undigested can damage the villi in your small intestines, thus preventing your ability to absorb even liquids. The human body has the capability of curing and healing anything if given enough time and proper fuel. See the first, second, and third golden rules of health above.

12. *Meat*: Organic chicken, turkey, or fish is allowed up to three times per week, and you can eat wild deer once a month. You need to eat meat sparingly, with little to no red meat and pork. Pork is the number one cause of parasites in the human body, which can cause cancer and other diseases. When eating meat, you will need extra hydrochloric acid and enzymes.

Dairy: You can use raw goat, Rice Dream, potato, carrot milk and almond milk. Raw cow's milk and seed nut's milk are also good. No homogenized or pasteurized milk! You can use raw butter in moderation, unsalted goat butter, or soy butter. You can also have goat or vegan cheese, yogurt, whey, cottage cheese, or cultured buttermilk but no American cheese, only hard cheeses. Seed and nut butters are good as well.

Egg: You can have organic eggs up to three times per week. They should not be fried but boiled soft for up to three minutes or poached. You can drink one raw egg yolk mixed with apple juice, two tablespoons of lecithin (or four capsules) every morning. You can also make this combination with black cherry juice and raw egg yolk.

Cooking oils: For cooking, you can use grape seed oil, which has the highest health benefits and smoke point, extra virgin olive oil and macadamia nut oil are okay but watch out for high temperature when cooking so the oil doesn't degenerate.

Water: At least six to eight glasses of water that was either purified or treated with reverse osmosis units, which are available at wholesale from NSP. A good rule to follow is to drink beyond your thirst. We should even drink up to one-ounce per one-pound of bodyweight during heavy detoxification. Drink little to no liquids with a meal. Instead, drink ten minutes before or one hour afterward. Liquids with a meal will dilute the digestive enzymes that our body manufactures.

Here are some additional suggestions given to our patients to keep them on health building program as they complete their treatments.

Important things to consider

HEALTHY APPROACH	TO AVOID
Suggested flours: rye, spelt or KAMUT flours, potato, rice, millet, buckwheat, amaranth	Whole wheat or gluten grains
	Refined sugar
Suggested sweeteners: Turbinado sugar, honey, maple syrup (in moderation), blackstrap molasses, licorice can be used as a sweetener and also stevia.	Root
	Alcohol and tobacco
	Black tea
Suggested beverages: caffeine-free herbal teas, green tea, coconut water and unsweetened fruit juices.	Coffee
	Soda pop
Suggested seasonings: Bragg's amino acid (good flavor, salty taste), veggie salt, sun-dried sea salt, Jensen's vegetable seasoning broth, Norwegian kelp, turmeric and red pepper (capsicum and cayenne)	Salt
	Pepper (black or white)

Health-building Juices	Quantity
- Carrot juice (straight) Optimal: half carrot juice and half goat's milk, pineapple juice, papaya juice, or apple juice.	Two 8-oz glasses per day

- Vital life juice
   - 2 oz carrots
   - 2 oz beets
   - 2 oz celery
Mix all together in a juicer.
	One glass per day

- Green cabbage drink	One 8-oz glass per day
- Grape juice	Up to 1 qt per day
- Raw liver - 2 oz mixed with 8 oz carrot juice	Once per week You can use organic liver, raw liver, or dissected raw liver capsules, which you can buy at any health food store.

Detoxification Rituals

ENEMAS	DAYS
Retention enemas should be held up to twenty minutes if possible.	Cold water causes contraction. Very warm water relaxes so you can retain longer.
COFFEE RETENTION ENEMAS - 8 oz of very warm water - 2 oz prepared teaspoons of coffee - 20 drops of peroxide (if using Oxy Toddy, use one capful per one oz).	Monday Wednesday Friday
SHARK RETENTION ENEMAS - 8 oz of very warm water - 2 tbsp. of shark powder	Tuesday Thursday

Regular Enema

There are many positions to take a regular enema. One of the best is on the knees-to-chest position, putting a towel underneath you to catch any spillage. A two-quart bag should be used and can be hung from a towel rack, or a hot-water bottle can be laid on a sink counter. Water should be five degrees warmer than body temperature. Water should be taken until you feel pressure. You should continue the enema until you can take all two quarts at one time and it comes out clean. Again, one ounce of flaxseed tea or bentonite should be used in water, and water should be filtered or passed through reverse osmosis for the best result. Remember, K-Y Jelly or calendula gel can be used as a sterile lubricant.

DETOX BATH - ¾ to 1 cup of pink sea salt - 1 tbsp. of baking soda - 3 tbsp. of ginger	DURING TREATMENT, WE RECOMMEND DETOX BATH DAILY: Too many baths in a day will weaken you. Staying in the tub too long will weaken you. Soaking for 14 minutes in a very hot tub of water once each day is sufficient. Make sure you wet your face, neck, and chest. Turn over in the tub if you can. If lightheaded or dizzy, place cold washcloths on head and back of neck. Be careful not to get a chill after the bath. Dry completely and cover up good.

Teas

Cuachalalate tea	1–4 cups per day
Pau d'arco tea	1–4 cups per day

What we have discovered is an individually prescribed program of therapies that can build up the immune system and destroy the invader cancer. These protocols greatly increase the chances of survival for cancer patients. Not only do they increase the survival rate, but they simultaneously enhance health, well-being, and quality of life after cancer.

Receiving calls from patients all over the world, we consistently find that patients cannot imagine a cancer treatment without surgery to start. We wanted to bring this science to you because we know that patients consider our treatment seriously, but only after having a medical procedure like surgery. We wanted to emphasize and make patients aware that right after their diagnosis, they can begin cancer treatment using immunotherapy and the protocols outlined in this book.

What we've found is using the immune system as part of the treatment is effective, combined with health-building strategies in the midst of the cancer battle. Our patients have been very impressed with the life-changing results created by these vaccines. We aren't making claims to reverse cancer one way or 100 percent of the time. No one as yet has discovered a single "magic bullet."

We hope you've enjoyed learning about immunotherapy and cancer vaccines that we believe are the backbone to breaking the cancer code. We visualize a future of breaking the cancer code. One that will shift the focus of reversing cancer, using methods that create an ideal cancer-fighting environment within the body, through enhanced immune system functioning. We hope this book helps patients and medical practitioners to make informed decisions with the power to heal.

Breaking the cancer code takes courage.
Courage is not the absence of fear; courage is the willingness to feel the fear and use your power to heal anyway.
Prevention is your willingness to change your lifestyle
and stay consistent with your health regimen no matter what.

Acknowledgments

Geronimo Rubio MD

My work would not be possible without the support of my entire family, *gracias por asu apoyo*. To my parents, Geronimo Rubio and Rebecca Guzman, I appreciate all your love and how proud you've been of my career as a doctor.

To my children: Geronimo Rubio Jr., MD, you have studied and worked with me as my right hand. I am so proud of your talent, helping me break the cancer code. Adrian, you have many bright and smart ideas to help the Rubio Cancer Center team with your psychology background. Irsa, you are my beautiful daughter and are supporting the oncology nutrition at the center. To my younger children, Yeroni and Yeraldine, I hope you become part of the family business. To my wife, Edena, you have supported me through the good times and bad times. I will never forget. Special thanks to my brother, Victor, for providing me with business strategy to help make the hospital grow.

Special thanks to Carolyn Gross, my patient advocate, for her tireless work in completing our book and Ramon, Consuelo, Michelle, Dianne, Rebecca, Sandra, Virginia, and the entire maintenance and kitchen staff.

A special thanks for my loyal staff for their many years of service:

Paulina Nunoz, RN, for twenty-six years; Dr. Barajas for twenty-three years; Dr. Patricia Smith, nineteen years; Mario Sierra for his nineteen years; and Dr. Herlinda Rivera for fourteen. Your spirits have helped shape Rubio Cancer Center to what it is today.

Dr. Livingston was an inspiration as an original researcher and honored me by being part of my first lectures. I have dedicated so much of my life to research, and her professional support helped me continue in my work.

Carolyn Gross

To my husband, Bryan, who has sacrificed so much of our time together so this book could be written. He is supportive and understands that I'm here to carry a message to others in need. My heart belongs to you!

To my father, the Kahuna, for always believing I was capable of doing great things!

This manuscript wouldn't have been polished and sensible without the help of Dr. Stephanie Henk and my longtime assistant Bao Phan. Thank you for your hard work and dedication.

My spiritual inspiration comes from many, so I always thank the *Book Angel* for the right people, stories, scenarios, and alliances to enhance my career and this book, including Dr. Patricia Smith, Sandra Orchin, Rev. Elizabeth Brabant, Barb Sanfilippo, Terry Jelley, Ce Ce Canton, Stacey Smith-Bacon, "Brother" Brooks, and the National Speakers Association.

Special thanks to the entire staff at Rubio Cancer Center and our amazing patients. Over the years, we've assisted many patients who were pastors, ministers, and game changers in their healing. Thank you for believing in our staff at Rubio Cancer Center. Thank you for our Amish and Mennonite patients as well for being so caring to everyone and sharing your faith-filled lives with us.

My special gratitude and honor goes to Geronimo Rubio MD. Thank you for saving my life and working together to save many more!

Resources

Bioelectrical Therapy

Biotele: Neurostimulation Technology Portal: *http://www.biotele.com/ bioelectric.htm*

Skyman: Bioelectrical World Without Pain: *http://www.21swd.com/en/ index.asp*

Cancer Treatment and Coaching Programs

Cancer Freedom Coaching Programs:

Creative Life Solutions
1081 Borden Rd. Suite 105
Escondido, CA 92026
Phone: 760.741.2762
Fax: 760.690.2352
Email: info@treatableandbeatable.com
http://www.breakingthecancercode.com
http://www.treatableandbeatable.com

Rubio Cancer Center
Granado NO. 420-A Fracc La Mesa
Tijuana, ME.C., Mexico 22440
Phone: 866.519.9960 or 760.294.0862
Email: info@rubiocancercenter.com
http://www.rubiocancercenter.com
http://www.cancerimmunologyrubiotreatment.com

Diet and Nutrition Web Sites

National Cancer Institute: *http://www.5aday.co.nz/*
Nutrition Cancer: *http://www.nutritioncancer.com/*
Nutritional Solutions: *http://www.nutritional-solutions.net/*

Guided Imagery

Academy for Guided Imagery: *http://acadgi.com/* ; 800-726-2070.
Guided Imagery Inc: *http://www.guidedimageryinc.com/*
Health Journeys: *http://www.healthjourneys.com/* 800-800-8661
The Healing Mind *http://thehealingmind.org/* ; 415-389-8941

Naturopathic Medical Schools/ Physician Associations and Referrals

American Association of Naturopathic Physicians:
http://naturopathic.org/content.asp?contentid=56

Association of Accredited Naturopathic Medical Colleges
http://www.aanmc.org/the-schools.php
818 18th Street NW, Suite 250
Washington, DC 20006
Phone: 202.470.6016
Fax: 206.299.9530
info@aanmc.org

Canadian Naturopathic Association
1255 Sheppard Avenue East
North York, Ontario M2K 1E2
Canada
416-496-8633
http://www.naturopathicassoc.ca

Naturopathy Online
http://www.naturopathyonline.com/

The American Association of Naturopathic Physicians
8201 Greensboro Drive, Suite 300
McLean, VA 22102
877-969-2267
http:// www.naturopathic.org

Psychoneuroimmunology

PsychoNeuroImmunology Research Society: http:// www.pnirs.org

The Norman Cousins Center for Psychoneuroimmunology (UCLA);
http://www.semel.ucla.edu/cousins
760 Westwood Plaza
Los Angeles, CA 90024
(310) 825-9989

The Peace Clinic: *http://the-peaceclinic.com/psycho-neuro-immunology-pni/*
The PsychoNeuroImmunology Research Society: http://www.pnirs.org
The Stress and Health Research Program at the Ohio State Medical
    Center: *http://pni.osumc.edu/default.htm*

Supplements

There are so many great products to recommend for cancer patients, that we
have specific referrals on our web site *www.breakingthecancercode.com*

Recommended Books

Bauman, Edward, MED, PhD, Waldman, Helayne, MS, EDD. *The Whole-Food Guide for Breast Cancer Survivors: A Nutritional Approach to Preventing Recurrence.* Oakland, CA: New Harbinger Publications Inc., 2012.

Bloom, William. *The Power of the New Spirituality: How to Live a Life of Compassion and Personal Fulfillment.* Wheaton, IL: Theosophical Publishing House, 2011.

Bogdanovich, Ruza, ND. *The Cure Is in the Cause: How You Can Eradicate Any Disease or Life Problem Once and for All, by Knowing the True Cause and Eliminating It.* Genoa, NV: Spirit Spring Foundation Inc., 2001.

Chic, Debra. *Secrets to Healing and Preventing Cancer: The First Complete, Total Health Program Built to Prevent, Inform and Guide People through Recovery from Cancer or Any Disease.* 2003.

Drost, Dan. *A Choice to Live: The Awesome Journey.* Tijuana, Mexico: ProMotion Publishing, 2010

Fitzgerald, Patricia, MD. *The Detox Solution: The Missing Link to Radiant Health, Abundant Energy, Ideal Weight, and Peace of Mind.* Santa Monica, CA: Illumination Press, 2001.

Gross, Carolyn. *Treatable and Beatable: Healing Cancer without Surgery.* Escondido, CA: Creative Living Publications, 2008.

Lee, Roberta, MD. *The Superstress Solution: Relieve Headaches and Anxiety. Sleep Well and Restore Your Ability to Relax. Control Your Weight. Build Resilience Against Future Stress.* New York, NY: Random House Inc., 2010.

Murray, Michael, MD. *How to Prevent and Treat Cancer with Natural Medicine: A Natural Arsenal of Disease-Fighting Tools for Prevention, Treatment, and Coping with Side Effects, from America's Foremost Authorities on Natural Medicine.* New York, NY: Riverhead Books, Penguin Putnam Inc., 2002.

Servan-Schreiber, David, MD, PhD. *Anticancer: A New Way of Life.* New York, NY: the Viking Press, 2008.

Ruzic, Neil. *Racing to a Cure*: *A Cancer Victim Refuses Chemotherapy and Finds Tomorrow's Cures in Today's Scientific Laboratories.* Chicago, IL: University of Illinois Press, 2003.

Mukherjee, Siddhartha. *The Emperor of All Maladies: A Biography of Cancer.* New York, NY: Scribner, a division of Simon & Schuster Inc., 2010.

Pond, David. *Chakras for Beginners: A Guide to Balancing Your Chakra Energies.* Woodbury, MN: Llewellyn Publications, 2011.

Galland, Leo, MD. *Power Healing*: *Use the New Integrated Medicine to Cure Yourself.* New York, NY: Random House Inc., 1998.

Phillips, Robert, PhD, Goldstein, Paula, CSW. *Coping with Breast Cancer: A Practical Guide to Understanding, Treating, and Living with Breast Cancer.* Garden City Park, NY: Avery Publishing Group, 1998.

Moss, Susan. *Keep Your Breasts!: Preventing Breast Cancer the Natural Way.* Los Angeles, CA: Re: Source Publications, 2002.

Diamond, John, MD, Cowden, Lee, MD, Goldberg, Burton. *An Alternative Medicine: Definitive Guide to Cancer.* Tiburon, CA: Future Medicine Publishing Inc., 1997.

Cunningham, Alastair, OC, PhD. *Can the Mind Heal Cancer?: A Clinician-Scientist Examines the Evidence.* www.HealingJourney.ca.

Williams, Xandria. *Vital Signs for Cancer Prevention: Protect Yourself from the Onset of Recurrence of Cancer.* Berkeley, CA: North Atlantic Books.

Lipton, Bruce, PhD. *The Biology of Belief: Unleashing the Power of Consciousness, Matter, & Miracles.* Carlsbad, CA: Hay House Inc., 2005.

Fuhrman, Joel, MD. *Eat for Health: Lose Weight, Keep It Off, Look Younger, Live Longer.* Flemington, NJ: Gift of Health Press, 2008.

Edwards Brothers Malloy
Thorofare, NJ USA
August 16, 2013